D1596105

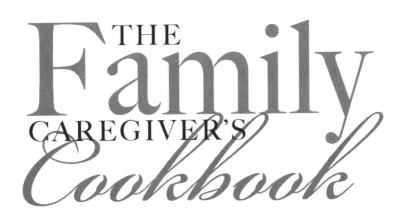

THE Family CAREGIVER'S Cookbook

Easy-Fix Recipes for Busy Family Caregivers

HARRIET HODGSON

Virginia

The Family Caregiver's Cookbook: Easy-Fix Recipes for Busy Family Caregivers

Copyright © 2016 by Harriet Hodgson. All rights reserved.

Published in the United States by WriteLife Publishing, Inc.

www.writelife.com

978-1-60808-160-8 (p)

978-1-60808-161-5 (e)

Library of Congress Control Number: 2016940178

Book design by Robin Krauss, www.bookformatters.com

Cover design by Ellis Dixon, www.ellisdixon.com

Cover photo and author photo by Haley Earley, Photographer

Frances Armstead, NDTR, RD, Nutrition Consultant

Harriet Hodgson's
The Family Caregiver Series

from WriteLife Publishing
www.writelife.com

The Family Caregiver's Guide: How to Care for a Loved One at Home

Affirmations for Family Caregivers

A Journal for Family Caregivers: A Place for Thoughts, Plans, and Dreams

The Family Caregiver's Cookbook: Easy-Fix Recipes for Busy Family Caregivers

Visit www.harriethodgson.com to learn more about this busy author, grandmother, and caregiver.

Visit www.thecaregiverspace.org/author/hhodgson to read her caregiving articles.

Acknowledgments

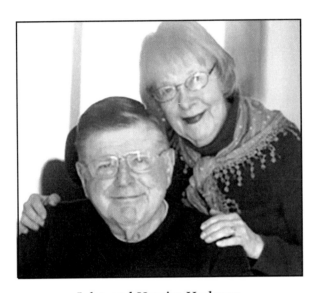

John and Harriet Hodgson

Photo courtesy of the *Post-Bulletin* newspaper, Rochester, MN, and P-B
photographer Elizabeth Nida Obert.

Thank you to nutrition consultant Frances Armstead for her appreciation of food and wise counsel.

Thank you to my granddaughter, Haley Earley, for her photography talents and technical help.

Thank you to Terri Leidich, President and Publisher of WriteLife Publishing, for believing in The Family Caregiver series. Although I've never met Terri, from working with her I can tell we are kindred souls.

Finally, thank you to my husband John, the inspiration for The Family Caregiver Series. You continue to amaze me and I love you more each day.

Contents

THE RECIPES

This book is written by a family caregiver for a family caregiver—**you.** The at-a-glance recipe format helps you prepare meals efficiently. All of the recipes in this collection are original. I have added healthy fruits and vegetables when possible. The sodium, sugar, and fat have been reduced without compromising on flavor. Icons help you find your way through the pages quickly. Here's a recipe map:

Recipe Title

Lead-In (personal story and/or information)
Prep Time (basics plus extra information)
Oven Temperature (if applicable)
Servings (normal size)
Ingredients (listed in order of use)
Method (includes bowl and pan sizes, cooking tools)
Caregiving Tips (from the author's on-the-job experience)

 A measuring cup marks the Ingredients section of the recipe.

 A whisk marks the Method section of the recipe.

A star marks the Caregiver Tips section of the recipe.

- Read the entire recipe before you start cooking.

- Save steps by gathering all the ingredients ahead of time.

- Make the recipes yours by changing the herbs, substituting ingredients, or adding a surprise ingredient.

Enjoy cooking healthy meals for your loved one and yourself!

PREFACE

The purpose of this cookbook is to help you prepare easy-fix, healthy food for the loved one in your care. It is based on my nineteen years of caregiving, decades of cooking, and love of food.

Although I'm not a professional chef, I was a food writer for the original *Rochester Magazine*, (when it started years ago in my hometown of Rochester, Minnesota), learned basic and advanced cooking techniques, and created many original recipes. I've made airy soufflés, gallons of soup, tossed a dizzying array of salads, baked French baguettes, turned our kitchen into a biscotti factory, produced thousands of cookies, made egg roll wrappers, flipped countless burgers, prepared a wedding dinner for seventy, roasted a Christmas prime rib as long as a log, entertained my physician husband's patients, and made cookbooks for family members.

These experiences have been a culinary journey, and I have enjoyed every moment of it—even the recipe failures.

I'm a "made-from-scratch" cook, an approach that halted abruptly in 2013 when my husband's aorta dissected. After three emergency operations, two months in the hospital, and six months in a nursing home for therapy, my husband John was released to my care. His dismissal was a nutrition wake-up call. For eight months I had been eating on the run. Instead of eating complete meals, I snacked and made poor food choices. Much as I hate to admit it, I often ate standing up due to time constraints. I visited my husband three times a day, at breakfast, lunch, and dinner, and there was little time for anything else.

While my husband was recovering, I moved us out of our three-story home, and built a wheelchair-friendly townhome for us. Visiting my husband, monitoring construction, and clearing out the home we lived in for more than twenty years stressed me as I had never been stressed before. I was running in all directions and my unhealthy diet became worse. Dinner was a bowl of cold cereal or ice cream. I took over many of John's tasks, ran the household, and managed our finances. Hurried and stressed, I often bought frozen meals and ate fast food—poor decisions for someone like me with high blood pressure. As the months passed, I realized I missed home cooking. Mixes and frozen meals have improved markedly, but they didn't taste homemade to me.

Your caregiving experiences may be similar to mine. After rushing to prepare food, using too many high-salt mixes, and eating too many frozen meals, many of them high in salt, you may yearn for something homemade.

Despite good intentions, you may not be able to follow through with your plans, and come up with excuses in self-defense. *I don't have enough time. The grocery store is so far away. My cooking skills are limited. I like to eat, but I don't like to cook. There isn't enough counter space. I don't have money for kitchen gadgets. Everything I make turns out weird. Why bother?*

My loved one doesn't like my cooking. These excuses may be true, yet they are manageable, and you can work around them.

After months of poor nutrition, I knew it was time to return to eating healthy, balanced meals. But finding the time to shop was a challenge and grocery shopping is a slow, demanding task for me. As a solution, I learned to plan far ahead, keep a well-stocked pantry, and speed shop for groceries.

I also learned that the approach to cooking by a caregiver requires taking a lot of things into consideration that we didn't have to think about before, including:

- physician's recommendations and prescriptions
- foods that inhibit or cancel effects of medication
- medication management (including dosage times)
- loved one's daily routine
- loved one's appetite
- food likes and dislikes
- amount of daily physical activity
- caregiving budget (including food)
- food intolerances and allergies

Challenging as my scenario was, these changes were possible, and I was willing to make them for my husband and me. I deserved balanced, nutritious meals as much as John, and getting back to normal eating would be comforting. John could hardly wait to eat a meal in his new home, and looked forward to eating his favorite foods, including marinated flank steak, six-inch-high popovers, all-beef meatloaf, salads with blue cheese, seasonal fruits, wine spaghetti sauce, and "anything with artichokes."

Relatives and friends offered to grocery shop for me, but I declined their offers. Grocery shopping was my field trip and I didn't want to give it up. Besides, I enjoyed seeing the seasonal produce, new products on store shelves, and chatting with friends. I've always been a list maker and my typed lists became more detailed. On the top half of the page I listed my daily "To-Do" points. On the bottom half of the page, I listed the groceries we needed, grouped according to the store layout: produce first, then bakery, meat, staples, cleaning supplies, and dairy.

This caregiver's cookbook is the result of my experience in providing nutritious meals for John and myself. While some recipes are based on existing ones, I've used them as a starting point only. Some ingredients were added, others were subtracted, methods and cooking times were changed, and I created new titles to grab your attention, and explain the recipes. My heart and soul are in this cookbook, as evidenced by the stories within these pages.

I've told you what this cookbook is, and need to tell you what it isn't. Since dozens of cookbooks have been published for people with food allergies, this cookbook doesn't contain recipes in this category. Many cookbooks have been published for those who have diabetes, so this cookbook doesn't contain recipes for diabetics. Diabetes is a complex disease, one that needs constant monitoring, and I think monitoring should be left to physicians, endocrinologists, and dietitians. Slow cooker cookbooks abound and, while some recipes give you the option of using a slow cooker, this cookbook isn't dedicated to it.

Frances Armstead, a nutrition consultant, helped me select the recipes, and checked them for health benefits. I'm grateful for her help and sensible approach to eating. Franny, as she likes to be called, believes all foods may be consumed in moderation. A marathon runner, she follows her own advice, is a made-from-scratch cook, watches her diet, and eats lots of fruits and vegetables. When I asked Franny, rather worriedly, if we should keep the recipes that contained whipped cream, she replied, "It's okay. You aren't eating whipped cream every day." Her reply made me want to cheer.

Most recipes tell which pan or bowl to use, a feature that Franny appreciates. Both of us read cookbooks the way some people read novels and we're fascinated by kitchen tools. Franny recommends testing the internal temperature of meat with an instant-read thermometer. You may wish to purchase this kind of thermometer if you don't have one. According to Mayo Clinic, the safe temperatures are: 150 F (74 C for any type of poultry, 160 F (71 C) for ground meat other than poultry, and 145 F (63 C) for solid cuts.

You don't need special equipment to make these recipes.

Basic supplies are all you need: different-sized pans/bowls, batter bowl (a large bowl with a handle and small spout), colander, sieve, cast-iron skillet, whisk, measuring cups/spoons, slotted spoon, wooden spoon, heat-resistant scraper, baking dishes, custard cups, serrated knife, paring/meat knives, and hand (immersion) blender. Discount and online stores carry these blenders and you can buy one for $18 and a few cents. I prefer a hand blender, as opposed to a stand blender, because it's safer, and I don't have to transfer hot liquids from pan to blender.

When I was writing these recipes I tried to imagine your caregiving day, the schedule you keep, and your time-management strategies. I tried to imagine the care receiver, too—a child with chronic disease, an ill husband or wife, or a grandparent in failing health. Every meal you prepare can exemplify the love you feel. Fixing meals for a loved one is more than providing fuel for the body; it's a demonstration of love. You can reduce salt and fat, monitor sugar, and avoid food additives, food coloring, and preservatives with unpronounceable names. Best of all, you can tailor the recipes to your loved one's needs.

Now turn the page, stock up, and start cooking!

STOCKING YOUR PANTRY

A well-stocked pantry saves you extra trips to the grocery store and reduces your stress. Put a checkmark by the items that are on your shelves. Keep in mind that herbs lose their flavor over time and some may need to be replaced. Your pantry may also include items your family likes and others that represent your heritage.

HERBS

- ○ Basil (dried)
- ○ Bay leaf
- ○ Cumin
- ○ Curry powder
- ○ Chili powder
- ○ Garlic
- ○ Ginger (dried and paste)
- ○ Italian blend or seasoning (a combination of parsley, oregano, basil, garlic powder, black pepper, marjoram, and onion flakes)
- ○ Marjoram
- ○ Onion powder
- ○ Oregano
- ○ Parsley (dried)
- ○ Poppy seeds
- ○ Rosemary
- ○ Sage

SPICES

- ○ Allspice
- ○ Black pepper
- ○ Cinnamon
- ○ Cloves
- ○ Dry mustard
- ○ Lemon pepper
- ○ Mace
- ○ Nutmeg (whole or ground)
- ○ Paprika (regular and smoked)
- ○ Seasoned pepper (a blend of black pepper, red bell peppers, sugar, and spices, without MSG)
- ○ Thyme

STAPLES

- ○ Almond extract
- ○ Artichokes (water packed)
- ○ Beans (canned and/or dried)
- ○ Beef broth (low sodium or no sodium)
- ○ Bouillon cubes (low sodium or no sodium)
- ○ Brown sugar
- ○ Chicken broth (low sodium or no sodium)
- ○ Cornstarch
- ○ Dijon mustard
- ○ Dried pasta (large and small)
- ○ Flour (all purpose)
- ○ Flour (quick mixing [Wondra])
- ○ Granulated sugar

- ○ Ketchup
- ○ Mayonnaise (reduced fat)
- ○ Olive oil
- ○ Orange extract
- ○ Pudding mixes (sugar free)
- ○ Rice (brown, white, and microwavable packs)
- ○ Red peppers (roasted and in a jar)
- ○ Salt
- ○ Soup (canned, reduced sodium)
- ○ Soy sauce (lower sodium)
- ○ Tomatoes (canned, reduced sodium or no sodium)
- ○ Tomato paste
- ○ Tomato sauce (no sodium)
- ○ Vegetable oil
- ○ Vinegar (different varieties)
- ○ Vanilla extract
- ○ Yellow mustard

SPEED SHOPPING TIPS

- Plan menus for a week and post them on the refrigerator.

- Keep a running list of the items you run out of.

- Avoid the 4:00–6:00 p.m. rush when grocery stores are crowded.

- To avoid parking problems and crowds, shop days before a national holiday.

- Become familiar with the store layout.

- Ask for a store directory. Large stores usually display them by the entrance or at the service counter.

- Shopping is generally faster when you make your list according to the store layout.

- Buy only the items on your list and resist impulse buying.

- Bring newspaper ads with you in case you can't find the specials and need to talk with a staff person.

- Look on low shelves for store brands (products distributed by the store, or with the store's name on them), which are generally cheaper than name brands.

- Don't assume that endcap items (displays on the end of shelves) are on sale. The supplier may have rented this space for more exposure.

- As you put things in your cart, group refrigerated/frozen items together.
- Group bread and bakery items together as well.
- Unload refrigerated and frozen food first and ask for them to be bagged together.
- Ask for ice cream to be bagged in plastic to slow melting.
- Separate meat from fresh produce.
- Ask for meat items to be bagged in plastic to avoid possible contamination.
- Ask for bakery items to be bagged together.
- Use coupons only if you have enough time. Check coupon expiration dates before you leave for the grocery store.
- Keep a cooler in your vehicle trunk for refrigerated/frozen items that have to be put away immediately.

Chapter 1

SOUP TODAY!

**Tomato-Basil Soup
with Shells
Page 16**

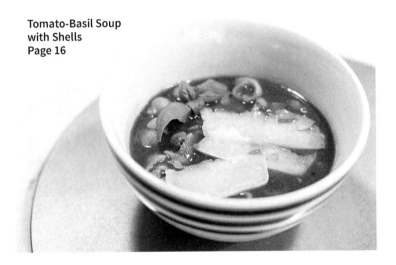

My love affair with soup began in elementary school when my mother made chowder with fresh clams. I can still see my father standing at the kitchen sink, helping her by opening clams with a small, scary knife. I enjoyed the chowder and really liked the little crackers on top. Soup is a smart meal decision for busy caregivers. You can make it days ahead, heat some when you need it, and freeze some for the future. Soup goes back centuries and the varieties are almost endless.

LEMONY ARTICHOKE SOUP

I created this recipe for a Christmas luncheon I hosted for friends. They loved the lemony soup and several friends asked for the recipe. While snow was blowing outside, inside we were warm, cozy, laughing, and slurping soup together.

Prep Time: 12 minutes + simmering
Servings: 12

Ingredients
3 cups tubettina pasta (tiny tubes), precooked
2 bags (8 ounces each) artichokes, frozen (or 2 cans [13.75 ounces each] artichokes, drained)
2 cartons (32 ounces each) chicken broth, salt free
2 chicken bouillon cubes
2 cups water
2 cups carrots, petite or baby (available in produce department)
3/4 cup Italian flat leaf parsley, chopped
1½ large lemons, juiced
Lemon pepper to taste
About 4 tablespoons flour (all-purpose or quick-mixing)
About 4 tablespoons cold water

Method

1. Cook pasta according to package instructions.
2. Defrost frozen artichokes in microwave. Cut large artichokes in half.
3. Combine chicken broth, bouillon cubes, water, artichokes, carrots, parsley, lemon juice, and lemon pepper in soup pot.
4. Bring to a boil, reduce heat, and simmer until carrots are tender, about 10 minutes.
5. Add cooked pasta.
6. Whisk flour into cold water, making sure there are no lumps, and slowly add to soup.
7. Cook over medium heat, stirring constantly, until soup thickens.

Caregiver Tips

You may make the entire recipe and freeze half for another day. I'm a big believer in the "another day" approach.

TOMATO-BASIL SOUP WITH SHELLS

This soup (pictured on the cover) is delicious, nutritious, and made with pantry staples. Serve it with French bread, hard rolls, or bread sticks.

Prep Time: 12 minutes + simmering
Servings: 8

Ingredients

2 tablespoons olive oil
1 yellow onion, chopped
1 carton (32 ounces) chicken broth, unsalted
1 can (28 ounces) tomato pureé
1 teaspoon garlic powder (more if you love garlic)
2 teaspoons sugar
1 teaspoon salt
1½ teaspoons dried basil (or 2 tablespoons fresh basil)
1/2 cup small-shell pasta (more if you're a noodle nut)
Parmesan cheese, shaved, for garnish

Method

1. Pour olive oil into soup pot. Sauté onions over medium heat for 5 minutes.
2. Add chicken stock, tomato pureé, garlic powder, sugar, and salt.
3. Cover and simmer for 5 minutes.
4. Add basil and small-shell pasta.
5. Cover and simmer until shells are cooked, about 10 minutes.
6. Garnish with shaved Parmesan cheese.

Caregiver Tips

Use pre-grated Parmesan cheese if you don't have a chunk of cheese. After it's refrigerated, the shell pasta continues to absorb moisture and you may have to add some more liquid before reheating it.

ROASTED RED PEPPER SOUP

This is a different and colorful soup. Vegetables make it healthy as well. You may pureé the soup with a hand blender, or eat it as is, with chunks of vegetables.

Prep Time: 15 minutes + simmering
Servings: 6 to 8

Ingredients

1 jar (15 ounces) roasted red peppers, drained and
     chopped
1 carton (32 ounces) chicken broth, salt free (or
     vegetable broth)
1 medium yellow onion, chopped
1 medium carrot, grated
1½ cups frozen hash browns
Black pepper to taste
Shredded Parmesan cheese, for garnish
Italian flat leaf parsley, for garnish

Method

1. Combine all ingredients, except cheese and parsley, in soup pot.
2. Bring to a boil, cover, and simmer for 15 minutes.
3. Pureé soup with a hand blender.
4. Ladle into bowls and garnish with shredded Parmesan cheese and snipped parsley.

Caregiver Tips

I use red peppers from a jar to save time. You may make your own roasted red peppers. Cut two red peppers into chunks, drizzle with olive oil, and roast in 400-degree oven until the peppers are tender and brown on the edges. The dark edges add extra flavor to the soup.

QUICK NEW ENGLAND CLAM "CHOWDAH"

John attended Dartmouth College in Hanover, New Hampshire, where the residents say "chowdah." Whenever I serve this to him, I say his "chowdah" is ready. He loves it. There is nothing quite like creamy New England Clam "Chowdah" for lunch or dinner.

Prep Time: 10 minutes + simmering
Servings: 4

Ingredients

2 strips bacon, cut into 1/2-inch pieces
1 can (18.5 ounces) New England Clam Chowder, light
1 can (6.5 ounces) chopped clams with juice
1/3 cup corn, frozen
Chowder crackers, for garnish

Method

1. Coat soup pot with cooking spray. Add bacon and cook over medium heat until brown.

2. Remove most of the bacon fat from pot.
3. Add chowder, clams, and corn.
4. Cover and cook over medium heat until corn is tender. Don't let this soup come to a boil.
5. Serve with chowder crackers.

Caregiver Tips

Some New England clam chowder recipes contain corn and others don't. Personally, I like the color and texture of the corn.

FIESTA MEXICANO SOUP

I make this soup with leftovers from the refrigerator: Spanish rice, salsa, a few vegetables, and a pound of ground beef. For flavor, I add a packet of taco seasoning. This soup is wonderful—a fiesta of flavors.

Prep Time: 15 minutes + simmering
Servings: 8 to 10

Ingredients

1 tablespoon olive oil
1 yellow onion, chopped
1 pound ground beef, 93% lean
1 cup carrots, chopped
1 cup celery, chopped
1 carton (32 ounces) chicken broth, no sodium
1 cup medium salsa
1 packet (1.25 ounces) taco seasoning, 40% less sodium
Half package (8.8 ounces) Spanish rice, microwavable
1 package (8 ounces) cheese product (like Velveeta)

Method

1. Pour 1 tablespoon of olive oil into soup pot. Add onion and cook for 4 minutes.
2. Crumble beef into pot and cook until brown.
3. Add carrots, celery, chicken broth, salsa, and taco seasoning.
4. Squeeze the rice packet to separate grains.
5. Add half of the rice to soup and refrigerate the rest for another time.
6. Cover soup and simmer for 15 minutes.
7. Cut cheese product into cubes and add to soup, stirring until cheese melts.
8. Serve with corn muffins or crusty bread.

Caregiver Tips

Add more salsa and cheese product if desired (the cheese product thickens the stock). I make this soup a day ahead, refrigerate it, and remove the fat from the top before I heat it again.

MUSHROOM-GINGER SOUP

Thanks to packaged, ready-to-use mushrooms, this is a quick, low-calorie soup. You can literally make it in minutes. Tiny carrots add color and flavor. I've served this soup to guests and they loved it.

Prep Time: 15 minutes + simmering
Servings: 6

Ingredients

2 tablespoons butter

1 carton (8 ounces) button mushrooms, cleaned and sliced

1 carton (8 ounces) baby Portobello mushrooms, cleaned and sliced

1/2 cup carrots, petite or baby (available in produce department), halved

1 carton (32 ounces) chicken broth (or vegetable stock)

1 tablespoon ginger paste

About 3 tablespoons cold water

About 3 tablespoons flour (all-purpose or quick-mixing)

Italian flat leaf parsley, chopped, for garnish

Method

1. Melt butter in soup pot. Add mushrooms and cook over medium heat until they start to brown, about 8 minutes.
2. Add carrots, chicken broth, and ginger paste.
3. Cover and cook over medium heat until carrots are tender, about 10 minutes.
4. Whisk cold water into flour, making sure there are no lumps. Slowly add mixture to soup and cook over medium heat, stirring constantly, until soup thickens.
5. Garnish with parsley.

Caregiver Tips

For cream of mushroom soup, add 1 cup half and half. If you like mushrooms, you'll enjoy this soup. Make it hours ahead and keep it warm in a slow cooker.

COWBOY CHILI WITH A JOLT OF JAVA

Cowboys helped settle the West. On long cattle drives, water was so valuable that the chuck wagon cook, called Cookie, saved coffee from one campsite to the next. Coffee was never thrown away and the pot was rarely washed. Grounds were added directly to the water. Cookie would add a beaten egg, even the shell, to the grounds to settle them to the bottom of the pot. When the grounds rose to the top, the coffee was done. Legend says the brew was so strong it could float a pistol, hence the name "Six Shooter" coffee. Extra coffee was sometimes added to recipes for a flavor, a cooking secret chefs still use today.

Prep Time: 20 minutes + simmering
Servings: 8

Ingredients

1 yellow onion, chopped
1 green pepper, chopped
1 red pepper, chopped
3 tablespoons olive oil
1½ pounds ground beef, 93% lean

1 can (14.5 ounces) diced tomatoes in juice, no salt

1 can (6 ounces) tomato paste, no salt

2 cups strong coffee

1 teaspoon salt

1 teaspoon smoked paprika

2 tablespoons chili powder (more if you like it hot)

1/2 teaspoon dried oregano

1 teaspoon garlic powder

1 can (14.5 ounces) kidney beans with juice (omit if you're allergic to beans, as I am)

Fat-free sour cream, for garnish

Low-fat Cheddar cheese, shredded, for garnish

Chopped avocado, for garnish

Method

1. Chop onion and peppers and set aside.
2. Pour 2 tablespoons olive oil into soup pot.
3. Cook beef over medium heat until brown.
4. Add onions and cook for 5 minutes.
5. Add remaining ingredients, cover, and simmer for 25 minutes.
6. Ladle into bowls and pass garnishes.

Caregiver Tips

Prepare the vegetables the day before, and finish the recipe the next day. Even if you're cooking for two, make the whole recipe. You'll have a ready-to-eat lunch or dinner for several days. This recipe may be simmered in a slow cooker.

MINNESOTA WILD RICE AND CHICKEN SOUP

Wild rice isn't rice at all; it's aquatic grass seed. My home state of Minnesota is the world leader in wild rice production. This grain contains more protein than wheat and is a good source of vitamin B. Because of its nutty flavor, you can reduce the salt in wild rice recipes. You may use wild rice for pilaf, soups, and salads. This recipe uses canned wild rice, a true time-saver.

Prep Time: 12 minutes + simmering
Servings: 8

Ingredients

1 tablespoon + 1 teaspoon butter

1½ tablespoons olive oil

1 box (8 ounces) button mushrooms, prewashed and sliced

1 can (15 ounces) wild rice, drained

2 cups rotisserie chicken, shredded (eliminate for vegetarian version)

Half package (6 ounces) carrots, petite or baby (available in produce department)

1/2 cup Italian flat leaf parsley, chopped

1 carton (32 ounces) chicken broth, no sodium (or vegetable broth)

2 chicken bouillon cubes (eliminate for vegetarian version)

1 can (10.5 ounces) mushroom soup, reduced sodium

2 soup cans water

1/4 cup sherry, very dry (optional), for garnish

Method

1. Melt butter and olive oil in soup pot.
2. Cook mushrooms over high heat until slightly brown.
3. Add all remaining ingredients.
4. Cover and simmer over low heat for 30 minutes.
5. Just before serving, add sherry to soup.

Caregiver Tips

Chopped ham or turkey may be substituted for the chicken. This recipe freezes well.

Chapter 2

FIVE-STAR SALADS

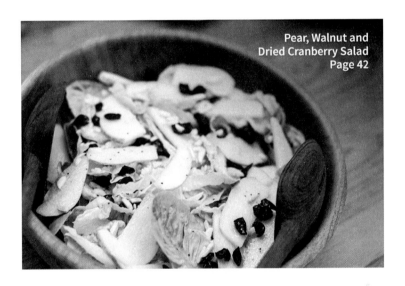

Pear, Walnut and
Dried Cranberry Salad
Page 42

I come from a family of salad nuts. In fact, the members of my family love salad so much, I fix twice the amount that "normal" people eat. When they were young, the three Hodgson brothers didn't like vegetables very much, but they would eat salad because it was crunchy, colorful, and fresh. After John and I married, I served him a variety of salads and started collecting recipes. The recipes in this chapter may make you a salad nut too.

CHINESE NOODLE SALAD WITH PEA PODS AND WALNUTS

I make this salad with wavy Chinese noodles because they cook in only three minutes. To make this recipe a main course, serve the salad with grilled chicken, shrimp, salmon, or steak. I think you'll agree that this salad is a winner!

Prep Time: 25 minutes
Servings: 8

Ingredients

1 package (10 ounces) Chinese noodles

1 cup walnut pieces, toasted, for garnish

1/2 cup bottled Asian dressing (fat free if available), plus extra dressing

1 red pepper, cut into thin strips

5 scallions, white and green parts, sliced diagonally

1 cup pea pods, halved, strings removed

1/2 cup carrots, shredded (from a package or shred them yourself)

1/2 cup fresh bean sprouts

1 package (6 ounces) fresh baby spinach

Method

1. Cook half the package of noodles in rapidly boiling water, separating them with a fork as they cook.
2. Rinse with cold water, drain, transfer to salad bowl, and cut into smaller pieces with kitchen scissors.
3. Toast walnuts in dry skillet until they start to brown. Cool on plate.
4. Toss noodles with 1/2 cup of Asian dressing.
5. Add vegetables (except spinach) and toss again.
6. Serve on top of fresh baby spinach and garnish with walnuts.
7. Pass extra dressing for those who want it.

Caregiver Tips

This salad may be eaten immediately or refrigerated for another time. Fresh bean sprouts keep only a few days, so use them quickly. Rice or whole-wheat noodles may be substituted for Chinese noodles.

SPINACH, ORANGE, AND AVOCADO SALAD

My husband loves the combination of citrus and avocado. Grapefruit segments may be substituted for orange segments. Use bottled dressing if you're pressed for time.

Prep Time: 20 minutes
Servings: 6

Ingredients
1 bag (6 ounces) baby spinach, stems removed
2 navel oranges, peeled and sectioned
2 avocados, sliced
2 scallions, white and green parts, chopped
2 tablespoons orange juice, frozen (thawed)
2 tablespoons white wine vinegar
2 tablespoons honey, more if you want a sweeter dressing
3/4 cup olive oil
1/2 teaspoon garlic powder (or 1 clove garlic, minced)
1/2 teaspoon salt (may be omitted)
1/4 teaspoon seasoned pepper
Chow mein noodles (optional), for garnish

Method

1. Pour spinach into salad bowl. Add orange sections, sliced avocados, and scallions.
2. Combine remaining ingredients (except chow mein noodles) in small jar. Put on lid and shake to combine.
3. Drizzle some dressing over the salad and toss. (Save the rest of the dressing for another time.)
4. Garnish with chow mein noodles if desired.

Caregiver Tips

For a really easy-fix recipe, use a small can of drained Mandarin oranges instead of fresh navel orange segments.

CHOPPED BLT SALAD WITH BLUE CHEESE

I first tasted this salad at a restaurant in the Mall of America in Bloomington, Minnesota. According to our server, the chopped salad is one of the restaurant's most popular dishes. The restaurant doesn't share recipes, so I paid close attention to the ingredients, amounts, and flavors. Although I wasn't able to estimate the exact measurements, this recipe tastes like the salad I enjoyed so much. This salad goes with almost everything.

Prep Time: 30 minutes
Servings: 6

Ingredients

1 cup small pasta, cooked (tubes, rings, or Acini di Pepe—little peppercorns)
1 teaspoon Dijon mustard
4 tablespoons olive oil
4 tablespoons rice vinegar
1/2 teaspoon salt
Coarsely ground black pepper to taste
1 package (2.5 ounces) real bacon pieces

3 large roma tomatoes, chopped
1 small bunch scallions, white and green parts, chopped
1/2 cup Blue cheese, crumbled
2 cups iceberg lettuce, chopped

Method

1. Cook pasta according to package instructions.
2. Rinse with cold water, drain, and transfer to salad bowl.
3. Put Dijon mustard, 4 tablespoons olive oil, rice vinegar, salt, and pepper in a small jar. Cover and shake to combine ingredients.
4. Add bacon pieces, tomatoes, scallions, blue cheese, and chopped lettuce to salad bowl.
5. Drizzle dressing over salad and toss well.

Caregiver Tips

You may use beefsteak tomatoes or quartered cherry tomatoes for this recipe. Cooked quinoa may be substituted for the pasta.

PEA AND CHEDDAR CHUNK SALAD

The deli in the grocery store I shop at makes a version of this salad, but it isn't as tasty or colorful as this one. To make this salad a main meal, serve it on lettuce leaves with shrimp, salmon, ham, or chicken.

Prep Time: 15 minutes
Servings: 6 to 8

Ingredients

2 cups frozen peas, rinsed under hot water and drained
1 rib celery, finely chopped
1/2 red pepper, finely chopped
2 hard-cooked eggs from the deli, chopped
2 scallions, white and green parts, chopped
4 ounces Cheddar cheese, (reduced fat, part skim), cubed
1/2 cup mayonnaise, light
1/2 cup slaw dressing, light

Method

1. Combine first six ingredients in salad bowl.
2. Stir mayonnaise and slaw dressing together.
3. Pour over salad and combine well.
4. You may eat this salad immediately or refrigerate it for later.

Caregiver Tips

Tempted as you may be, don't use canned peas for this recipe. Canned peas don't look or taste the same as frozen ones.

BEEFSTEAK TOMATO AND FETA SALAD WITH FRESH BASIL

Simple is often better and this recipe illustrates that point. The combination of tomatoes and fresh basil is classic. This attractive salad tastes especially good with Italian food.

Prep Time: 10 minutes
Servings: 4

Ingredients

4 lettuce leaves
3 large beefsteak tomatoes, sliced
4 tablespoons salad olives with pimientos, drained
4 tablespoons feta cheese, reduced fat
6 basil leaves, cut into strips with kitchen shears, for garnish

Method

1. Get four small plates. Place one lettuce leaf on each plate.
2. Put 2 slices of tomato on each leaf and top with 1 tablespoon of salad olives.
3. Sprinkle 1 tablespoon of feta cheese over the olives and garnish with basil.
4. Finish with salad dressing on page 37.

Caregiver Tips

This is an easy and attractive salad to make. It tastes best when made with summer tomatoes.

PEAR, WALNUT, AND DRIED CRANBERRY SALAD

Fresh pears and toasted walnuts seem to be made for each other. Bottled raspberry dressing may be substituted for homemade.

Prep Time: 12 minutes
Servings: 6

Ingredients

2 heads little lettuce hearts (miniature lettuce heads in a package—you may use other kinds of lettuce if the little hearts aren't available)
1/3 cup walnut pieces, toasted in dry skillet, for garnish
1 teaspoon yellow mustard
4 tablespoons olive oil
4 tablespoons cider vinegar
1 tablespoon honey
1/2 teaspoon salt
Coarse ground black pepper to taste
1 Anjou pear, unpeeled, thinly sliced
1/4 cup dried cranberries, with 50% less sugar

Method

1. Separate leaves on little lettuces and place in salad bowl.
2. Toast walnuts in dry skillet over low heat, stirring several times, until they start to brown. Cool on plate.
3. Put yellow mustard, olive oil, vinegar, honey, salt, and pepper in a jar. Cover and shake to combine.
4. Scatter pear slices and dried cranberries over lettuce.
5. Drizzle dressing over salad and garnish with toasted walnuts.

Caregiver Tips

Some people are allergic to walnuts, so ask family members and guests about their allergies before you make this recipe. Sliced almonds may be substituted for walnuts. You may garnish this salad with Roquefort or blue cheese.

MIXED GREENS WITH LEMON AND OREGANO VINAIGRETTE

The lemon juice and oregano in this recipe turn leafy greens into a special salad. You may use bottled dressing if you're short on time, but homemade dressing saves you money.

Prep Time: 15 minutes
Servings: 6 to 8

Ingredients

1 head butter lettuce (or Boston), torn into small pieces
1/2 head red leaf lettuce, torn into small pieces
1 small bunch of watercress (or lettuce)
1 teaspoon Country Dijon mustard
1/3 cup olive oil
1/3 cup fresh lemon juice
1/4 teaspoon garlic powder
1/2 teaspoon dried oregano
1/4 teaspoon salt
1/4 teaspoon lemon pepper
Packaged garlic croutons, or reduced-salt croutons, for
    garnish

Method

1. Put washed lettuces and watercress in a salad bowl.
2. Combine mustard, olive oil, lemon juice, garlic, oregano, salt, and lemon pepper in a jar.
3. Cover and shake to combine.
4. Drizzle some dressing over salad and toss gently.
5. Garnish with croutons.

Caregiver Tips

This salad is an ideal match for chicken or fish dishes. Double the dressing recipe so you have some for another day.

LETTUCE WEDGE WITH ROQUEFORT CRUMBLE DRESSING

When John and I were first married, lettuce wedge salad topped with dressing made with mayonnaise, ketchup, and pickle relish was popular. Lettuce wedge salad is popular again. Many restaurants serve it topped with Roquefort dressing, bacon, and tomatoes, but it's pricey. Don't pay restaurant prices for this side dish. Be budget-wise and make your own!

Prep Time: 15 minutes
Servings: 4

Ingredients
1 medium-sized head iceberg lettuce, cut into four
    wedges
1 cup mayonnaise, light
1 carton (8 ounces) sour cream, fat free
1/2 cup buttermilk, low fat
1 teaspoon Worcestershire sauce
Roquefort cheese (as much as you want)

1 package (2.5 ounces) real bacon pieces, warmed, for garnish

4 cherry tomatoes, halved, for garnish

Method

1. Place lettuce wedges on individual plates.
2. Gently combine mayonnaise, sour cream, buttermilk, Worcestershire sauce, and Roquefort in a bowl.
3. Spoon over lettuce.
4. Garnish with crumbled bacon and tomatoes.

Caregiver Tips

Blue cheese may be substituted for the Roquefort. I buy a wedge of Danish cheese for this recipe and crumble it myself. This dressing also tastes good on hamburgers; just omit the buttermilk.

SWEET CARROT SALAD WITH BLUEBERRIES

This is a welcome change to the old-fashioned shredded carrot and raisin salad. While the old-fashioned recipe is good, I think this one is better. The orange carrots and dark berries make this salad visually appealing.

Prep Time: 15 minutes
Servings: 8

Ingredients
2 packages (16 ounces each) raw carrot chips
2 tablespoons water
Bowl of ice water
4 scallions, white and green parts, cut diagonally
1 rib celery, cut diagonally
1/2 cup fresh blueberries
2 limes, zested and juiced
1 teaspoon Dijon mustard
2 tablespoons olive oil
2 tablespoons honey
1/4 teaspoon salt

Method

1. Put carrots in microwave-safe bowl. Add 2 tablespoons water and cook on high for 5 minutes, or until crisp tender.
2. Rinse in ice water to stop cooking and drain.
3. Transfer to salad bowl. Add scallions, celery, and blueberries.
4. Zest and juice limes over jar. Add Dijon mustard, olive oil, honey, and salt. Cover and shake to combine.
5. Drizzle over salad and toss.

Caregiver Tips

Dried cranberries or sliced apricots may be substituted for blueberries. Although you can use bottled dressing if you're short on time, don't use a tomato-based dressing because it won't taste very good with the fruit.

MUFFULETTA-STYLE PASTA SALAD

New Orleans, Louisiana is famous for many foods—chicory coffee, sugary doughnuts, and the Muffuletta sandwich. This sandwich is stacked with hard salami, ham, Provolone cheese, and olive relish, a flavorful combination. I combined these flavors in a main-dish salad and wrote an article about it that included the recipe. Months later, while I was surfing the Internet, I came across my recipe on a restaurant menu.

Prep Time: 20 minutes + boiling
Servings: 6

Ingredients
2 cups whole-wheat rotini, cooked
1 cup green pepper, chopped
1 cup red pepper, chopped
1 cup carrots, shredded, from a bag
1/2 cup salad olives with pimientos
1/3 cup celery, chopped
3 tablespoons Italian flat leaf parsley, chopped
2 tablespoons Kalamata olives, halved
5 slices hard salami, julienned

2 slices Provolone cheese, julienned
Bottled Italian dressing

Method

1. Cook rotini according to package instructions. Rinse with cold water, drain, and transfer to salad bowl.
2. Add remaining ingredients to bowl, drizzle with Italian dressing, and toss well.
3. You may eat the salad immediately or refrigerate for later.

Caregiver Tips

This salad keeps well and tastes even better the next day.

Chapter 3

MEAT MAGIC

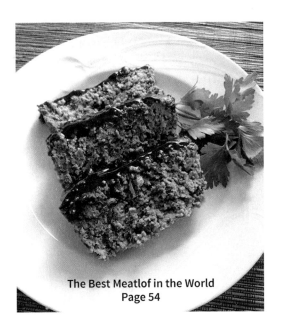

The Best Meatlof in the World
Page 54

In honor of my British heritage I usually make roast beef and Yorkshire pudding for Christmas dinner. One year the roast was done earlier than expected. To keep our Golden Retriever from eating it, I covered the roast with foil, and set it on top of the car in our garage. Family members smelled the roast the instant they walked in the door. "Is that dinner?" my sister-in-law asked. I answered affirmatively. Two years later Christmas was at our house again. When my sister-in-law walked into the house she asked, "Is dinner on top of the car this year?" It wasn't, but the memory made us smile.

THE BEST MEATLOAF IN THE WORLD

My mother-in-law gave me this recipe. We like it because it's made with only beef and has a sweet topping. Although we've enjoyed other meatloaf recipes, we like this one the most, and think it's the best meatloaf in the world. You won't want to waste a crumb of this satisfying recipe. I've even made meatloaf pizza!

Prep Time: 15 minutes + baking
Oven Temperature: 350 degrees
Servings: 6

Ingredients

2/3 cup wheat bread crumbs (or 1/3 cup Panko bread crumbs)
1 cup fat-free milk
2 large eggs, beaten
1/2 yellow onion, grated (or 1 teaspoon onion powder)
1 teaspoon salt
1/8 teaspoon pepper
1/2 teaspoon sage
1½ pounds ground beef, 90% lean
1/2 cup ketchup

3 tablespoons dark brown sugar
1 teaspoon dry mustard (or 1 teaspoon Dijon mustard)
1/8 teaspoon nutmeg

Method

1. Heat oven to 350 degrees.
2. Coat meatloaf pan with cooking spray.
3. Put bread crumbs, milk, eggs, onion, salt, pepper, and sage in a batter bowl. Combine with whisk.
4. Using a fork, gently work ground beef into milk-egg mixture.
5. Transfer to prepared pan.
6. In a small bowl, stir ketchup, brown sugar, mustard, and nutmeg together. Spread evenly over top of meatloaf.
7. Bake 1 hour.
8. Let meatloaf rest for a few minutes before slicing.

Caregiver Tips

One day I didn't have an onion on hand, so I added half of a 2.9-ounce can of French-fried onions to the meat. Since fried onions are salty, I added half a teaspoon of salt instead of a whole teaspoon. Use leftover meatloaf for sandwiches, crumble into spaghetti sauce, or add to vegetable soup.

EASY SWEDISH MEATBALLS

I'm originally from Great Neck, Long Island, New York. Our next-door neighbors, Esther and Axel, came from St. Paul, Minnesota. "Aunty Esther" introduced me to Swedish Meatballs and I loved them. Still do. But I have to admit that her tiny meatballs were better than mine. Every meatball was made with love and tasted like it. Whether it's dinner or lunch the next day, Swedish meatballs are a favorite at our house.

Prep Time: 15 minutes + baking
Oven Temperature: 350 degrees
Servings: 5 to 6

Ingredients
1¼ pounds ground beef, 93% lean
1/3 cup onion, minced (or 1 teaspoon onion powder)
1 large egg, beaten
1/2 cup fat-free milk
1/3 cup Panko bread crumbs
1 teaspoon salt (may be omitted)
2½ teaspoons sugar
1/2 teaspoon allspice

1/4 teaspoon nutmeg + dash for meatball topping
1 can (10.5 ounces) mushroom soup, reduced salt
1 soup can water
1 beef bouillon cube
Mashed potatoes, rice, or cooked noodles

Method

1. Heat oven to 350 degrees.
2. Coat a rimmed pan and casserole dish with cooking spray.
3. Combine first nine ingredients in a large bowl.
4. Form into small balls, set in pan, and bake for 15 minutes.
5. Transfer to prepared casserole.
6. Combine mushroom soup, water, bouillon cube, and nutmeg in bowl. Pour over meatballs and bake 1 hour.
7. Serve over mashed potatoes, rice, or noodles.

Caregiver Tips

Canned soup is the time-saver in this recipe. The meatballs should be about the size of a quarter. You could make the meatballs a day ahead, and finish the recipe the next day. Swedish Meatballs may also be cooked on low in a slow cooker for 4 hours.

COFFEE RUB FOR MEAT

Meat rubs add additional flavor and this gives you a chance to cut back on salt. Coffee, garlic, and brown sugar give this rub its flavor. Dark brown sugar helps the meat to brown.

Prep Time: 10 minutes + resting and grilling
Servings: 8

Ingredients
1 teaspoon instant coffee (or unbrewed, ground coffee)
2 teaspoons garlic powder
1 teaspoon ground dry mustard
1 teaspoon smoked paprika
2 teaspoons dark brown sugar
2 teaspoons salt
1/2 teaspoon seasoned pepper
Olive oil (to drizzle over meat)

Method
1. Combine all ingredients (except olive oil) in small

bowl, making sure there are no lumps.
2. Rub into pork chops, steak, chicken, or hamburgers.
3. Let rub rest for 10 minutes.
4. Drizzle meat with olive oil and grill.

Caregiver Tips

You may wish to double this recipe and store it in a tightly sealed container for future use. Eliminate salt if necessary.

CUBE STEAKS WITH ROQUEFORT SAUCE

Cube steaks used to be called minute steaks and for a good reason; they take only minutes to cook. The sauce in this recipe enhances the flavor of the beef. Serve with mashed potatoes, rice, or cooked orzo.

Prep Time: 25 minutes + simmering
Servings: 4

Ingredients

4 beef cube steaks
Flour for dredging meat
1 tablespoon olive oil
1 tablespoon butter
1½ cups beef broth, salt free
1 teaspoon salt (may be omitted)
Freshly ground black pepper to taste
Dash garlic powder
1/2 cup Roquefort cheese, crumbled
1 teaspoon ketchup
1 tablespoon cornstarch
1 tablespoon cold water

Method

1. Dredge steaks in flour.
2. Put olive oil and butter in skillet. Heat until butter has melted.
3. Add steaks and cook over medium heat until both sides are golden brown.
4. Remove steaks from skillet, set on plate, and cover with foil.
5. Add beef broth, seasonings, Roquefort cheese, and ketchup to skillet.
6. Whisk cornstarch and water together, making sure there are no lumps. Add to sauce and cook over medium heat, stirring constantly, until sauce thickens.
7. Return steaks to skillet and simmer, uncovered, for 10 minutes.

Caregiver Tips

Cut overly large cube steaks in half. If you're not a Roquefort fan, delete it from this recipe. The steaks and sauce will still taste good.

BEEF BURGUNDY

The original recipe for Beef Burgundy (Boeuf Bourguignon), a fragrant stew, comes from France. I've made Julia Child's recipe many times. It's incredibly delicious and labor-intensive. My recipe takes less time and the orange zest adds freshness to the stew.

Prep Time: 20 minutes + simmering
Servings: 4

Ingredients

1 tablespoon olive oil
1 tablespoon butter
1¼ pounds beef stew meat, cut into 1-inch pieces
1 package (2.5 ounces) real bacon pieces, precooked
Half box (4 ounces) button mushrooms, cleaned and
    sliced
1/2 yellow onion, chopped
2 cups Burgundy (red wine)
2 tablespoons tomato paste, no salt
1 cup water
2 beef bouillon cubes
1 bay leaf

1 cup carrots, petite or baby (available from produce
    department)
1 tablespoon orange zest
2 tablespoons flour, quick-mixing
2 tablespoons cold water

Method

1. Put oil and butter in Dutch oven.
2. As soon as butter has melted, add beef, and cook over medium heat until brown and crusty.
3. Add remaining ingredients, except flour and cold water. Cover and simmer 1 hour.
4. Whisk cold water into flour, making sure there are no lumps. Slowly add to stew and cook over medium heat, stirring constantly, until sauce has thickened.
5. Serve over mashed potatoes, rice, or noodles.

Caregiver Tips

This recipe may be finished in a slow cooker. Cook on high 1 hour, turn to low, and cook 4 more hours. Cabernet may be substituted for Burgundy.

TERIYAKI SKEWERS

When I ask family members to tell me their favorite meal, they usually say "teriyaki." Although you can broil skewers in the oven, charcoal grilling is the best method. The brown sugar in this marinade gives the meat a flavorful crust. My family members think homemade marinade tastes better than the bottled kind.

Prep Time: 15 minutes + marinating and grilling
Servings: 4

Ingredients

1/2 cup light soy sauce
2 tablespoons dark brown sugar
2 tablespoons olive oil
1/4 teaspoon seasoned pepper
1 teaspoon garlic powder
1½ pounds sirloin steak, cut into 1-inch cubes (or 1½ pounds pork tenderloin)

Method

1. Combine marinade ingredients in a large bowl.
2. Add meat, cover, and marinate at room temperature for 2 hours.
3. Thread meat onto skewers.
4. Grill over hot coals for 10–12 minutes, turning several times, and basting with marinade.
5. Watch carefully. You want the meat to brown, not burn.

Caregiver Tips

Use this marinade for whole steaks too. You may make separate vegetable kabobs to go with the beef: onion pieces, red pepper, green pepper, and whole water chestnuts. Serve with plain rice or fried rice.

BEEF PICADILLO WITH MEXICAN RICE

Picadillo is a South American or Spanish dish usually made with ground beef. This recipe uses the last of a beef roast. I buy top-round roasts when they are on sale and we get several meals from one. This recipe uses leftover beef in a creative, delicious way.

Prep Time: 20 minutes + simmering
Servings: 4

Ingredients

1 tablespoon olive oil
1 yellow onion, chopped
1 green pepper, chopped
2 cups leftover roast beef, cut into small cubes
1 can (8 ounces) tomato sauce
1/2 cup salad olives with pimientos
1/2 cup raisins (dark or golden)
Water if needed
1 package Mexican rice mix (weight varies; buy the brand that seems best)

Method

1. Coat bottom of skillet with 1 tablespoon olive oil.
2. Add chopped onion and cook for 3 minutes.
3. Add green pepper and cook until soft.
4. Add remaining ingredients (except water and rice).
5. Cover and simmer over low heat for 20 minutes to blend flavors.
6. Add a little water if the mixture is too thick.
7. Prepare rice as directed.
8. Spoon sauce over rice.

Caregiver Tips

If the roast is a less tender cut, simmering is a good way to tenderize the meat. This recipe tastes just as good with ground beef.

LAMB BURGERS A LA ATHENS

Several years ago my husband and I went to Athens, Greece. We enjoyed many meals in the Old Town section of the city. Stray dogs eyed our meals and they scared me a bit. Would a dog run up to the table and eat my food? Thankfully, that didn't happen. These burgers remind me of Greek food, and go well with a Greek salad.

Prep Time: 15 minutes + frying
Servings: 5 to 6

Ingredients

1 pound ground lamb
1/3 cup Panko bread crumbs
1 large egg, beaten
1/2 cup feta cheese, reduced salt
1 tablespoon Italian flat leaf parsley, chopped
1 teaspoon garlic powder
1 teaspoon oregano
1 teaspoon salt
2 teaspoons lemon zest, grated
1/2 teaspoon lemon pepper

Method

1. Combine all ingredients in a large bowl.
2. Form into thin patties.
3. Cook in skillet until no longer pink inside.
4. Place on hamburger buns or insert into pita bread.

Caregiver Tips

Some stores mix ground beef with ground lamb. This recipe tastes best with just lamb. The meat mixture may be formed into small meatballs, browned in a skillet, and stuffed into pita bread with lettuce, tomatoes, and cucumber slices (a gyros sandwich).

GLAZED PORK TENDERLOIN

Pork tenderloin is a delicious, low-fat meat, and often on sale. I buy tenderloins that are just over a pound. We eat a third of the meat, and I use the rest for stir-fry and barbecued pork sandwiches.

Prep Time: 15 minutes + roasting
Oven Temperature: 350 degrees
Servings: 4

Ingredients

1 pound pork tenderloin
1 small bunch scallions, left whole
2 tablespoons Dijon mustard
1/2 cup reduced-sugar peach or apricot marmalade

Method

1. Heat oven to 350 degrees.
2. Cover bottom of baking pan with nonstick foil.
3. Cut tenderloin in half horizontally.
4. Insert whole scallions and close meat.

5. Mix mustard and marmalade together. Frost the top of the tenderloin with this mixture.
6. Insert a few toothpicks into tenderloin to hold it together.
7. Roast meat for 45 minutes, or until done.

Caregiver Tips

Tempted as you may be, don't use yellow mustard for this recipe because the flavor just won't be the same.

LITTLE BEEF OR PORK SLIDERS

These sliders are packed with flavor. Form the mixture into six big burgers if you wish. These sliders taste best when they are charcoal grilled.

Prep Time: 15 minutes + grilling or frying
Servings: 6

Ingredients
1 can (8 ounces) water chestnuts, finely chopped
1/3 cup Panko bread crumbs
1½ pounds ground beef, 85% lean (or 1½ pounds ground
  pork)
2 scallions, white and green parts, finely chopped
1/4 cup soy sauce, reduced sodium
1½ teaspoons ginger paste
1 teaspoon garlic powder
2 tablespoons dark brown sugar
Seasoned pepper to taste
12 small buns
Lettuce (optional), for garnish
Light mayonnaise (optional), for garnish
Sweet and sour sauce (optional), for garnish

Ketchup (optional), for garnish
Sliced avocado (optional), for garnish

Method

1. In a large bowl combine all ingredients, except buns. Mix gently with fork.
2. Form into 12 small patties.
3. Charcoal grill or cook in skillet.
4. Transfer to buns and serve with accompaniments.

Caregiver Tips

Make the burgers several hours ahead of time. You may also form the burgers and freeze them.

CENTER-CUT HAM SLICE WITH CITRUS SAUCE

A ham slice exemplifies an easy-fix meal. Before you buy a center-cut slice, check the water content on the label. Some brands are 25 percent water! Choose the brand with the least amount of water. I often buy small, thick-cut, reduced-sodium ham slices for this recipe.

Prep Time: 15 minutes + simmering
Servings: 4 to 5

Ingredients

1 center-cut ham slice
1/2 cup barbecue sauce (pick the brand with the least salt)
1/4 cup marmalade, sugar free
1/4 cup orange juice (fresh or frozen)

Method

1. Coat skillet with cooking spray.
2. Add ham and brown both sides.

3. Transfer to plate and cut into serving-sized pieces.
4. Add barbecue sauce, marmalade, and orange juice to skillet.
5. Simmer for about 8 minutes to combine flavors.
6. Return ham to skillet and simmer until ham is hot.
7. Serve with choice of sides.

Caregiver Tips

You may make this recipe with presliced ham from the meat department or deli.

HEAVENLY WINE SPAGHETTI

Feeding a crowd? This is the recipe to make. Decades ago, I found this recipe in a magazine and cut it out. But the recipe was lost during one of our many moves, and now I make it from memory. Of course I altered the recipe to suit our tastes. We love, love, love this sauce! Once you've tried it, I think you will like it as much as we do.

Prep Time: 25 minutes + simmering
Servings: 12

Ingredients

1 pound pork sausage, reduced fat
2 pounds ground beef, 93% lean
4 yellow onions, chopped
4 to 5 cloves of garlic, minced in press (or 3 teaspoons garlic powder)
1 cup fresh Italian flat leaf parsley, chopped
2 cans (15 ounces each) tomato sauce, no salt
Half bottle (normal size) dry red wine of your choice
3 teaspoons Italian blend seasoning
Cooked spaghetti or soba noodles

Method

1. Brown sausage in skillet and remove with slotted spoon.
2. Brown ground beef in same skillet and remove with slotted spoon.
3. Put onions, garlic, parsley, tomato sauce, wine, and Italian blend in soup pot. Turn heat to high and boil for 5 minutes to cook off alcohol.
4. Add cooked meat to pot. Cover and simmer on lowest heat for 2 hours.

Caregiver Tips

To feed a smaller group, make half the recipe. You may make the sauce in advance and freeze it.

GRILLED STEAK TOPPED WITH HERB BUTTER

We invited a Texas couple for dinner. Menu: beef tenderloin, wild rice pilaf, green salad, and a fancy dessert. I cut the meat into medallions, and cooked them in a smoking hot skillet. Each person received two medallions topped with herb butter. "What's this?" the husband asked, pointing to the meat. Since we had lived in the Lone Star State, we knew folks ate steaks big as dinner plates. "Beef tenderloin," I replied. The husband nodded, started eating, and said little. Was dinner a flop? At the end, the husband exclaimed, "That was as good as a Texas steak!"

Prep Time: 15 minutes + chilling and frying
Servings: 8

Ingredients

2 tablespoons Italian flat leaf parsley, minced
2 teaspoons chives, finely chopped
2 teaspoons tarragon, minced
1/2 teaspoon garlic powder
1/2 teaspoon salt
1/2 teaspoon seasoned pepper

1 stick of butter, room temperature
Your choice of steak

Method

1. Stir ingredients (except steak) together in a medium bowl, making sure the herbs are combined well.
2. Cover bowl and chill butter 1 hour.
3. Coat skillet with cooking spray. Fry steak until medium. Don't judge doneness by color. Check internal temperature with instant-read thermometer.
4. Top each serving of meat with herb butter just before serving. (I cut orbs of butter with a melon baller.)

Caregiver Tips

Herbed butter also tastes great on grilled hamburgers, chicken, or fish. This compound butter keeps for about a week in the refrigerator.

Chapter 4

FISH AND SHELLFISH

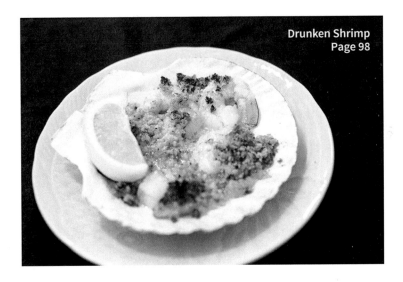

Drunken Shrimp
Page 98

Fish is good for you according to a Mayo Clinic article, *Omega-3 in Fish: How Eating Fish Helps Your Heart.* "Fatty fish, such as salmon, lake trout, herring, sardines and tuna, contain the most omega-3 fatty acids," the article notes. These acids can have several health benefits, including decreasing triglycerides, and lowering blood pressure and the risk of heart failure and stroke. We try to eat fish once a week (although I falter sometimes) and because we live in the Midwest, it's usually frozen or canned. If fresh fish is readily available where you live, enjoy it!

DEVILED CRAB IN SHELLS

Can you make a can of crab taste good? You bet. This recipe is delicious and appealing. I bake the crab in individual scallop shells that I bought in San Francisco years ago. You may bake the crab in individual, oven-proof dishes.

Prep Time: 15 minutes + baking
Oven Temperature: 350 degrees
Servings: 2

Ingredients

1 tablespoon butter
1 rounded tablespoon flour, quick-mixing
3/4 cup fat-free milk
1/8 teaspoon lemon pepper
1/2 teaspoon sugar
Dash each paprika and nutmeg
1 egg, beaten
1 tablespoon lemon juice
2 tablespoons pimientos, chopped
1 teaspoon dried parsley flakes
1 can (6 ounces) fancy lump crabmeat (or fresh crabmeat)

2 tablespoons olive oil
1/2 cup Italian bread crumbs

Method

1. Heat oven to 350 degrees. Coat 2 small baking dishes with cooking spray.
2. Melt butter in saucepan.
3. Add flour and cook 1 minute.
4. Whisk in milk, lemon pepper, sugar, paprika, and nutmeg. Cook over medium heat, stirring constantly, until sauce thickens.
5. Stir 1 tablespoon of this mixture into beaten egg.
6. Add egg mixture, lemon juice, pimientos, and parsley to saucepan. Cook 1 minute and remove from heat.
7. Fold crabmeat into sauce and spoon into dishes.
8. Combine olive oil and bread crumbs and sprinkle over crab.
9. Set dishes on baking sheet and bake for 25–30 minutes, until crab starts to bubble around the edges.

Caregiver Tips

This recipe may be doubled or tripled and baked in a casserole dish. Serve with crusty bread and a green salad.

MEXICAN FISH AND VEGETABLE PACKETS

Sole is an adaptable fish and you can make it taste the way you want. Green chiles, chili powder, cumin, and salsa make this fish flavorful. Red pepper and corn add color. Serve this fish with Mexican rice and a salad.

Prep Time: 15 minutes + baking
Oven Temperature: 400 degrees
Servings: 4

Ingredients

1 pound sole fillets (or wild-caught Alaskan cod)
1 teaspoon chili powder
1 teaspoon cumin
1 can (7 ounces) fire-roasted green chiles
1 small onion, halved and cut into crescents
1 red pepper, sliced into strips
1 cup corn, frozen, unthawed
1 cup salsa of your choice
4 slices Monterey Jack cheese, reduced fat

Method

1. Heat oven to 400 degrees. Tear 4 large squares of nonstick foil from roll. Coat each one with cooking spray.
2. Place an equal amount of fish on each square.
3. Sprinkle with chili powder and cumin.
4. Drain green chiles and cut into smaller pieces.
5. Layer onion, some chiles (you won't need them all), red pepper, and corn over fish.
6. Layer salsa evenly over fish and place slices of cheese on top.
7. Fold opposite sides of foil once, leaving enough interior space for steam to escape, and fold again. Crimp ends of packets.
8. Set packets on jelly roll pan and bake for 20 minutes.

Caregiver Tips

Boy Scouts and Girl Scouts have been making foil meals for years. Easy clean-up and versatility are the pluses of this recipe. You can use any vegetables you have on hand, such as zucchini or mushrooms. This is an easy recipe to make for a crowd. Assemble the packets an hour ahead and refrigerate until mealtime.

CRISPY COD WITH POTATO CHIP TOPPING

This recipe gives you the texture of fried fish without the frying. The preparation is super-easy. You coat the fish with a combination of crushed potato chips, Italian bread crumbs, and crackers, and bake it. About twelve minutes later, you're sitting down to dinner!

Prep Time: 12 minutes + baking
Oven Temperature: 375 degrees
Servings: 4

Ingredients

3/4 cup reduced-salt potato chips, finely crushed
1/3 cup crackers, crushed (about 5)
1/2 cup Italian bread crumbs
2 tablespoons butter, melted
8 to 10 ounces wild-caught Alaskan cod fillets
Cooking spray, to coat tops of cod fillets

Method

1. Heat oven to 375 degrees. Coat baking pan with cooking spray.
2. Put potato chips and crackers in plastic zipper bag. Seal bag and crush contents with rolling pin.
3. Add Italian bread crumbs and combine with spoon.
4. Transfer crumb mixture to pie plate and stir in melted butter.
5. Place fillets on baking pan.
6. Coat top of fillets with cooking spray so crumbs will stick.
7. Sprinkle some crumbs on top of each fillet.
8. Bake for 12–15 minutes, or until fish flakes with a fork, yet is moist.

Caregiver Tips

Use plain potato chips for this recipe, not the flavored kind, which will overpower the fish. Don't over bake the cod, or it will become dry.

CONFETTI TUNA

I think it's reassuring to have a can of tuna on the shelf. This recipe turns canned tuna into a delicious salad, sandwich filling, topping for mixed greens, or crostini. Confetti Tuna is packed with calcium, has some crunch, and lots of flavor.

Prep Time: 15 minutes
Servings: 8

Ingredients

1 can (7 ounces) water-packed tuna, drained
1 cup cottage cheese, fat free
2 hard-cooked eggs, chopped (available from the deli)
2 roma tomatoes, chopped
2 tablespoons pickle relish
1/2 cup celery, diced
1 cup Cheddar cheese, reduced fat, shredded
1/2 cup mayonnaise, light
1 teaspoon lemon juice
1/2 teaspoon lemon pepper

Method

1. Flake tuna into large bowl.
2. Add remaining ingredients and mix gently with fork.
3. You may eat the salad immediately or chill it for later.

Caregiver Tips

If you use this salad for sandwiches, add extra crunch with iceberg lettuce, romaine lettuce, or alfalfa sprouts.

GRILLED SESAME SALMON

Grilling is one of the easiest ways to cook salmon. You may use a charcoal grill, gas grill, or cast-iron grill pan. Watch for sales on salmon because many grocery stores have them.

Prep Time: 15 minutes + marinating and grilling
Servings: 4

Ingredients

1/4 cup sesame seeds, toasted, for garnish
1 large orange, zested and juiced (zest for garnish)
1/2 cup rice vinegar
3 tablespoons pure maple syrup (not light or sugar free, which won't caramelize properly)
4 salmon fillets (about 4 to 6 ounces each)
Extra maple syrup, for garnish

Method

1. Toast sesame seeds in a dry skillet until they start to brown, about 5–8 minutes. Remove from skillet and set aside.

2. Zest the orange. Place zest in a small bowl and cover with plastic wrap.

3. Squeeze orange and put juice in a plastic zipper bag. Add vinegar and pure maple syrup to bag. Stir with spoon to combine.

4. Add fish, seal the bag, and marinate for 3 hours.

5. Coat grill with cooking spray.

6. Place fish on grill and frequently baste with marinade. Cook about 4 minutes per side. Fish is done when it flakes with a fork.

7. Remove from grill and drizzle each fillet with maple syrup.

8. Garnish with sesame seeds and orange zest.

Caregiver Tips

Black sesame seeds, or a combination of white and black, may be used for this recipe.

BAY SCALLOPS AND GARLIC PASTA

Scallops are one of my favorite foods, but the large ones are expensive. Bay scallops are cheaper and when I see them on sale, I can't resist them. I made up this recipe on the spur of the moment and, if I say so myself, it's fantastic!

Prep Time: 20 minutes
Servings: 5 to 6

Ingredients

12 ounces thin spaghetti (or soba noodles)
2 tablespoons butter (no substitutions)
1 pint bay scallops with liquid
1 roasted red pepper from a jar, drained and chopped
3 tablespoons Italian flat leaf parsley, chopped
2 tablespoons garlic bread spread (from the spice section of the store)
Lemon pepper to taste
2 tablespoons dry white wine, or pasta water
Shredded Parmesan cheese, for garnish

Method

1. Cook spaghetti until al dente—tender but not totally cooked. Rinse with cold water, drain, and transfer to bowl.
2. Coat large skillet with cooking spray.
3. Melt butter in skillet.
4. Add scallops and their liquid. Cook over medium heat until scallops are opaque. Do not overcook!
5. Add roasted red pepper, parsley, garlic spread, lemon pepper, and wine (or pasta water) to scallops.
6. Incorporate spaghetti with this mixture. Cover and simmer 2 minutes.
7. Spoon into individual bowls and garnish with Parmesan cheese.

Caregiver Tips

Scallop liquid is a key component of this recipe and infuses the spaghetti with flavor. The liquid is so delicious you'll want to sop it up with bread.

TANGY SALMON BURGERS

I created this recipe with leftover salmon from a restaurant meal and the burgers were really good. John liked them more than the original salmon, and that's saying something. This recipe uses canned salmon. Make sure the label contains the word "wild," which differs from farm-raised salmon. Serve burgers on a bun with lettuce and tomato or plain with lemon and tartar sauce.

Prep Time: 15 minutes + frying
Servings: 4 to 5

Ingredients
1 can (16 ounces) wild salmon
1/4 cup Panko bread crumbs
2 large eggs, beaten
1/4 cup Italian flat leaf parsley, chopped
2 tablespoons red onion, minced
1 tablespoon lemon zest
2 tablespoons lemon juice
1/2 teaspoon lemon pepper
1 tablespoon olive oil

Buns

Lettuce, tomato, mayonnaise, lemon, tartar sauce (for garnish)

Method

1. Drain salmon and flake into large bowl.
2. Add bread crumbs, eggs, parsley, onion, lemon zest, juice, and lemon. Mix gently with fork.
3. Form into 6 burgers.
4. Put 1 tablespoon oil in skillet. Cook burgers on both sides until they start to brown.
5. Serve on buns with lettuce, tomato, and mayonnaise, or lemon and tartar sauce.

Caregiver Tips

Italian bread crumbs may be substituted for Panko crumbs. You may add lemon juice to the mayonnaise for a flavor punch.

SHRIMP AND PASTA DELIGHT

Artichokes, tomatoes, and shrimp are a marvelous combination of flavors. Use your favorite pasta in this recipe—spaghetti, angel hair, linguini, rotini—whatever suits your budget and palate.

Prep Time: 12 minutes + sautéing
Servings: 4

Ingredients
Half box (8 ounces) spaghetti or soba noodles
3/4 pound shrimp, frozen with tails on
2 lemons, zested and juiced
2 tablespoons butter
1 cup artichokes, frozen, defrosted, and halved
1/2 teaspoon lemon pepper
1 chicken bouillon cube
1/2 cup water
1 tablespoon olive oil
1 cup roma tomatoes, chopped
1/2 cup Italian flat leaf parsley, chopped, for garnish

Method

1. Cook spaghetti according to package directions.
2. Rinse with cold water, drain, and transfer to bowl.
3. Defrost shrimp according to package directions and remove tails.
4. Zest and juice lemons. Set juice and zest aside separately.
5. Pour olive oil into skillet. Add butter, shrimp, lemon juice, artichokes, lemon pepper, bouillon cube, and water. Cook 2 minutes.
6. Add pasta, lemon zest, and tomatoes. Toss with tongs to distribute ingredients.
7. Garnish with parsley.

Caregiver Tips

I keep frozen shrimp on hand because it's such a time-saver. You may use fresh shrimp if you wish.

DRUNKEN SHRIMP

I make individual servings of this dish, but you may prefer a casserole. This recipe takes only minutes to prepare and bakes for only a few minutes. What an easy-fix meal!

Prep Time: 15 minutes + baking
Oven Temperature: 350 degrees
Servings: 4

Ingredients
2 pounds shrimp, frozen with tails on
4 tablespoons butter
1 teaspoon garlic powder
1/3 cup Italian flat leaf parsley, chopped
1/3 cup sherry, dry (or cooking sherry)
1/4 teaspoon lemon pepper
2 tablespoons olive oil
1 cup Italian bread crumbs

Method

1. Heat oven to 350 degrees. Coat a small casserole dish with cooking spray.
2. Defrost shrimp according to package directions and remove tails.
3. Put butter and garlic powder in microwavable measuring cup. Cover with plastic wrap to contain spatters and heat in microwave about 1 minute, or until butter melts.
4. Remove from microwave and add parsley, sherry, and lemon pepper.
5. Arrange one layer of shrimp in casserole dish and drizzle with butter-sherry mixture.
6. Combine olive oil and bread crumbs and scatter over shrimp.
7. Bake 10 minutes, or until crumbs start to brown.

Caregiver Tips

I serve this recipe with rice pilaf, baked potatoes, and orzo mixed with peas. Add a green salad and you have a wonderful meal.

HOLIDAY OYSTER STEW

Oyster stew is a centuries-old recipe. *The Boston Cooking School Cook Book* by Fannie Merritt Farmer, first published in 1896, contains a recipe for it. Many modern cookbooks have the same recipe—oysters warmed in milk and butter. Eating oyster stew on Christmas Eve is our family tradition. I add red pepper, chopped parsley, and paprika for color. Our daughters responded to oyster stew with "yuk" when they were little. As the years passed, "yuk" became "yum." First they tried a piece of oyster, a whole oyster, and finally the stew.

Prep Time: 15 minutes + warming
Servings: 4

Ingredients
1 pint raw oysters, shucked, with liquid
1/4 cup butter
1 tablespoon Worcestershire sauce
1 teaspoon celery salt
1/8 teaspoon freshly ground black pepper
1/2 teaspoon paprika
1 quart whole milk

1½ tablespoons red pepper, minced
1 tablespoon Italian flat leaf parsley, chopped
Oyster crackers, for garnish

Method

1. Check oysters for bits of shell.
2. In a soup pot, melt butter until it starts to sizzle.
3. Add oysters and their liquid, Worcestershire sauce, celery salt, pepper, and paprika. Cook over low heat until edges of oysters start to curl.
4. Add milk, red pepper, and parsley.
5. Warm over medium heat, but do not boil.
6. Garnish with oyster crackers.

Caregiver Tips

I don't add extra salt to this recipe because the oysters, Worcestershire sauce, celery salt, and oyster crackers (if used) are enough.

Chapter 5

ADAPTABLE EGGS

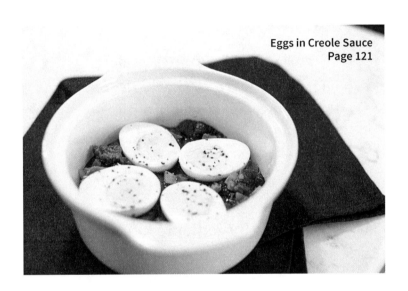

Eggs in Creole Sauce
Page 121

Eggs are budget friendly and you can cook them in many ways. We like cheese soufflé and I've made different versions: Cheddar, Roquefort, mushroom, broccoli. In one of our former homes the stove was next to the garage door. If the door slammed the stove shook, so I posted a note for my husband. It read: "DO NOT SLAM DOOR. SOUFFLE IN OVEN!" John fondly remembers these notes.

MINI BREAKFAST PIZZAS

These mini pizzas will wake you up and make you eager for a new day. Kids and grandkids may help assemble the pizzas.

Prep Time: 15 minutes + baking
Oven Temperature: 400 degrees
Servings: 6

Ingredients

1 six-pack English muffins (regular, whole wheat, or sourdough)
1 teaspoon butter
6 large button mushrooms, thinly sliced
1½ cups egg substitute (or 6 eggs, beaten)
2 tablespoons scallions, chopped
1 jar (25 ounces) Alfredo sauce, light
1 package (16 ounces) ham, chopped
1½ cups gruyere cheese (or Swiss cheese), shredded

Method

1. Heat oven to 400 degrees.
2. Separate sliced muffin tops and bottoms with fork. Set on rimmed baking pan.
3. Toast muffins in oven for about 8 minutes. Remove from oven.
4. Melt butter in a nonstick skillet.
5. Cook mushrooms until they start to brown. Transfer mushrooms to small bowl.
6. Pour egg substitute (or beaten eggs) into skillet and add scallions. Cook over medium heat, stirring several times with a heat-proof scraper, until eggs start to set.
7. Transfer egg-scallion mixture to another bowl.
8. Spoon some Alfredo sauce onto each muffin half. Top with a few sliced mushrooms, chopped ham, scrambled egg substitute, and gruyere or Swiss cheese.
9. Bake for 10–12 minutes, or until cheese has melted.

Caregiver Tips

For color, add some chopped roasted red peppers from a jar. Make extra mini pizzas if you have teenagers or young adults in the house.

RED PEPPER, ONION, AND MUSHROOM FRITTATA

This is one of the fastest egg dishes you can make. Frittata is partially cooked on a stovetop and finished in the oven. Cooking experts recommend a nonstick, oven-proof skillet for frittatas. Since I don't have one of those skillets, I cook vegetables in my cast-iron skillet, transfer them to a pie plate, add the egg mixture, and bake until set.

Prep Time: 20 minutes + baking
Oven Temperature: 375 degrees
Servings: 8

Ingredients

1 tablespoon olive oil
1 small red pepper, chopped
1 yellow onion, chopped
Half a box (4 ounces) mushrooms, cleaned and sliced
2 tablespoons Italian flat leaf parsley, chopped
1 teaspoon dried thyme
Salt and pepper to taste
8 large eggs (or 4 eggs, and 1/2 cup egg substitute)

1/4 cup fat-free milk

3/4 cup Mozzarella cheese, reduced fat, shredded

Method

1. Heat oven to 375 degrees. Coat a pie plate with cooking spray.
2. Pour olive oil into skillet. Add vegetables (except parsley) and cook, stirring several times, until crisp tender.
3. Add parsley and seasonings. Transfer vegetables to pie plate.
4. In a medium bowl, whisk eggs, milk, and cheese together. Pour over vegetables, making sure the egg mixture reaches the bottom of the plate.
5. Set plate on cookie sheet. Bake until set, about 35–45 minutes.
6. Cut into wedges.

Caregiver Tips

Experiment with different vegetables, such as baby spinach and grated zucchini. You may also try different cheeses.

CHICKEN AND MUSHROOM CREPES

Crepes sound intimidating, but they are just pancakes. You may use crepes for savory or sweet dishes. Years ago, I made lasagna with crepes that I cut into strips, and it was excellent. My younger daughter talks about the crepe lasagna to this day.

Prep Time: 12 minutes + resting and cooking
Oven Temperature: 325 degrees
Servings: 12

Ingredients

3 large eggs, room temperature
1¾ fat-free milk
1/2 teaspoon salt
2/3 cup all-purpose flour
1/2 cup butter, melted, plus additional melted butter for skillet
1 can (10.5 ounces) cream of chicken soup, reduced salt
Half soup can fat-free milk
2 cups rotisserie chicken, chopped
3 tablespoons celery, chopped
3 tablespoons pimientos, chopped

Dash soy sauce
1/2 cup almonds, sliced, for garnish

Method

1. Whisk eggs, milk, and salt together. Slowly add flour, whisking until lump-free.
2. Whisk in butter.
3. Cover bowl and refrigerate for 2 hours.
4. Brush sides of a 7-inch, nonstick skillet with melted butter.
5. Pour 1/4 cup batter into skillet and tilt to distribute batter. Cook batter over low heat until set, and bottom is light brown.
6. Using a heat-proof scraper, flip crepe over and cook 1 minute.
7. Transfer to wax paper. Do not stack crepes.
8. Place half of the soup in a medium saucepan. Add half soup can of milk, chicken, celery, pimientos, soy sauce, and heat until warm.
9. Spoon a little sauce onto each crepe, roll, and set in baking dish seam side down.
10. Pour remaining soup over crepes, garnish with almonds, and bake for 20 minutes.

Caregiver Tips

Make the crepes ahead of time and freeze with wax paper between each one. Use store-bought crepes if you're pressed for time.

SWEET, SOOTHING CUSTARD

A loved one without much appetite may be willing to eat custard. Bake this recipe in a casserole dish or individual custard cups.

Prep Time: 15 minutes + baking and refrigeration
Oven Temperature: 350 degrees
Servings: 6

Ingredients
Boiling water to pour into rimmed baking pan
3 large eggs, room temperature, slightly beaten
1/4 cup granulated sugar
1/8 teaspoon salt
1 teaspoon pure vanilla extract
1/4 teaspoon pure almond extract
2½ cups whole milk (or 2%)
Dash nutmeg
Whipped cream or topping (may be omitted), for garnish

Method

1. Heat oven to 350 degrees.
2. Boil some water in a kettle or pan.
3. In a large bowl, whisk eggs, sugar, salt, and extracts together. Stir in milk.
4. Pour into 6 ungreased custard cups or a 1½-quart casserole dish and sprinkle with nutmeg.
5. Set cups in a 13" x 9" rimmed baking pan.
6. Pour 1 inch of boiling water into the pan, being careful not to get any into cups.
7. Set pan on center oven rack and bake for 45 minutes, or until a paring knife comes out clean.
8. Refrigerate until set.
9. Serve with whipped cream or topping.

Caregiver Tips

Instead of whipped cream, scatter a few sliced strawberries or raspberries on top of the custard.

FRIED RICE WITH SCRAMBLED EGGS

This recipe comes together in minutes. For convenience and health, I use microwavable brown rice and egg substitute. You may use leftover cold rice instead.

Prep Time: 15 minutes
Servings: 4

Ingredients

1/2 cup egg substitute, scrambled (or 2 large eggs, scrambled)

1 tablespoon vegetable oil

2 scallions, white and green parts, sliced diagonally

1 package (8.8 ounces) microwavable brown rice, cooked according to package instructions

1 cup mixed frozen peas and carrots (or frozen mixed vegetables)

Soy sauce (lower sodium), to taste, plus extra sauce for garnish

Method

1. Coat a small skillet and large skillet with cooking spray.
2. Scramble egg substitute (or 2 eggs) in small skillet and set aside.
3. Pour vegetable oil into large skillet and cook scallions for 1 minute.
4. Cut scrambled eggs into chunks. Add to large skillet, along with rice and vegetables, and stir-fry 2–3 minutes.
5. Season lightly with soy sauce and stir.
6. Serve immediately.

Caregiver Tips

This recipe is a nice side dish for pork chops, pork tenderloin, teriyaki-marinated steak, or burgers.

BUONGIORNO EGGS AND SPAGHETTI

Whenever I cook pasta, I cook extra for future meals. Originally, this recipe was a way for Italians to use up leftover spaghetti. Somewhere I read that the pasta omelet is a popular lunch in Naples, Italy. I don't remember where I read this, but I've been to Italy, and savored the food. Enjoy this dish for any meal and pretend you are there.

Prep Time: 15 minutes
Servings: 2 to 4

Ingredients

1 can (8 ounces) tomato sauce, no salt (or 1 cup marinara sauce)

1 tablespoon butter

2 cups plain spaghetti, cold, cut into small pieces

1 carton (16 ounces) egg substitute (or 4 eggs, beaten)

2 tablespoons Parmesan-Romano cheese, grated, plus extra for garnish

Salt and pepper to taste

Method

1. Pour tomato or marinara sauce into small pan and set over low heat.
2. Melt butter in 8-inch, nonstick skillet.
3. Put a layer of cut spaghetti (1/2–3/4 cup) in skillet.
4. Pour just enough egg substitute or beaten eggs over spaghetti to cover pasta.
5. Cook over medium heat, pushing mixture to the center and letting uncooked eggs run to side, several times.
6. Sprinkle with Parmesan-Romano cheese and season with salt and pepper.
7. Using two spatulas, flip "pancake" over and cook other side for 1 minute.
8. Slide onto serving plate.
9. Repeat this process again.
10. Top spaghetti discs with sauce and pass more Parmesan-Romano cheese.

Caregiver Tips

For color, you may wish to add some chopped Italian parsley to the egg-spaghetti mixture. If you don't want to eat tomato sauce for breakfast, omit it.

CURRIED EGG SALAD WITH CASHEWS

Eggs and curry go together well. The cashews add an elegant touch to ordinary egg salad. You may eat this as a salad, or over lettuce, served with tomatoes and cucumber on top, or as a sandwich filling.

Prep Time: 12 minutes
Servings: 4

Ingredients

4 eggs, hard-cooked, available from the deli
1/2 cup celery, diced
2 scallions, white and green parts, finely chopped
1/2 cup cashew pieces, salted
1/3 cup mayonnaise, light
1 teaspoon curry powder
1 tablespoon fresh lemon juice
1/2 teaspoon salt
Freshly ground black pepper (optional), for garnish

Method

1. Combine all ingredients in large bowl.
2. Add ground black pepper if you wish.

Caregiver Tips

This salad is best when eaten immediately. If you make it too far ahead the cashews lose their crunch. I like this salad on whole-wheat bread, or on crackers for a quick snack.

BACON AND CHEESE STRATA

This mock soufflé is easy to make. You cut bread slices into cubes, layer the cubes in a baking dish with bacon and cheese, pour a mixture of milk and eggs over everything, and bake the strata. Eggs, bacon, and cheese are an unbeatable combination.

Prep Time: 15 minutes + baking
Oven Temperature: 350 degrees
Servings: 6

Ingredients

8 pieces wheat bread, crusts removed, cut into cubes

8 pieces precooked bacon, crumbled

1½ cups Cheddar cheese, reduced fat, shredded (more if you wish)

3 large eggs, room temperature, plus 1/2 cup egg substitute

1½ cups fat-free milk

1 teaspoon Dijon mustard

Method

1. Coat baking dish with cooking spray, and scatter a layer of bread cubes in the bottom.
2. Sprinkle with bacon and cheese.
3. Add a second layer to dish, ending with cheese.
4. In a batter bowl, whisk eggs, milk, and mustard together. Pour over bread and let stand 1/2 hour.
5. Heat oven to 350 degrees.
6. Set dish on middle oven rack and bake, uncovered, for 45 minutes, or until the cheese has melted and the top is puffy and golden.

Caregiver Tips

Because bread, bacon, and cheese are salty, there is no salt in this recipe. Save time by using packaged bacon. This dish tastes good when made with a Mexican cheese blend, Colby-Jack cheese, or if you're adventuresome, Pepper Jack.

EGGS IN CREOLE SAUCE

I first tasted this dish in a Shrafft's Restaurant in New York City. Although this restaurant chain is gone now, my memory of this tasty lunch remains. My friend and I ordered Creole eggs because they were one of the cheapest items on the menu. We were surprised at how delicious they were, and enjoyed every morsel. This is my version of that memorable luncheon.

Prep Time: 18 minutes + heating
Servings: 4

Ingredients

2 tablespoons olive oil
1 tablespoon butter
1 yellow onion, chopped
1 green pepper, chopped
1 teaspoon garlic powder
1/2 teaspoon smoked paprika
1/8 teaspoon dried rosemary
1 can (14.5 ounces) petite cut tomatoes in juice
Dash hot sauce
8 hard-cooked eggs, halved, available from the deli

Method

1. Put olive oil and butter in skillet.
2. As soon as butter has melted, add onion, green pepper, garlic powder, smoked paprika, and rosemary.
3. Cook 5 minutes.
4. Combine canned tomatoes with vegetables.
5. Set eggs in sauce. Add a little water if necessary. Cover and simmer 5 minutes, or until eggs are hot.
6. Serve eggs and sauce over rice, or with a hard roll.
7. Pass hot sauce if desired.

Caregiver Tips

You may use deviled eggs for this recipe.

PASTRY BREAD PUDDING

I'm originally from Great Neck, Long Island, New York. There was a Jewish bakery in the heart of the village and its baked goods were legendary. My mother often sent Dad to the bakery to buy a package of buns or coffee cake. Dad couldn't resist the coffee cakes and bought one, two, or three. He would walk in the door and announce the total sheepishly. Some pastries became stale, and Mom made bread pudding with them. Finding fruits and nuts in the bread pudding made me feel like I was on a treasure hunt.

Prep Time: 12 minutes + baking
Oven Temperature: 325 degrees
Servings: 8

Ingredients

Boiling water to pour into large pan
3 cups whole milk
2 large eggs, room temperature
1/3 cup granulated sugar
1 teaspoon pure vanilla extract
1/2 teaspoon salt (may be omitted)

3 cups stale pastry (Danish, cinnamon rolls, coffee cake),
   cut into 1-inch cubes
Whipped cream or sugar-free whipped topping, for
   garnish

Method

1. Heat oven to 325 degrees.
2. Coat baking dish with cooking spray.
3. Boil some water in a small saucepan.
4. Heat milk in large saucepan until bubbles appear.
5. In a medium bowl, whisk eggs, sugar, vanilla extract,
   and salt together.
6. Gradually whisk egg mixture into milk.
7. Add pastry cubes to milk and pour into baking dish.
8. Set dish in a large baking pan. Pour boiling water into
   pan until it comes halfway up the dish.
9. Bake 1 hour, or until knife comes out clean.
10. Serve warm with whipped cream.

Caregiver Tips

Use freshly whipped or aerosol cream for this recipe.
Recently I read an article about making bread pudding
with doughnuts. I won't be doing that because it is the

pastry that gives this bread pudding its flavor. Doughnuts could have been cooked in old oil, which could spoil the dessert.

Chapter 6

POULTRY DISHES

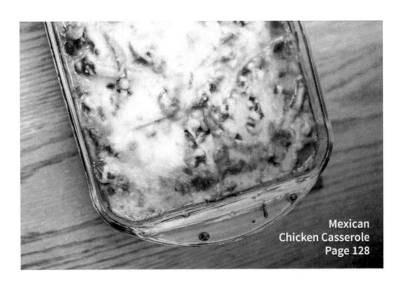

Mexican
Chicken Casserole
Page 128

Chicken cooks quickly and accepts many flavors: mushroom, garlic, Parmesan cheese, tomato, chili, soy sauce, and more, as well as ethnic seasonings, such as Jamaican Jerk. Grocery stores often have sales on chicken, so watch for them. Buying chicken on sale gives you the opportunity to make a double recipe, freeze the extra, or deliver a meal to another caregiver. Boned rotisserie chicken may be used for some of these recipes.

MEXICAN CHICKEN CASSEROLE

Cooking is easy when you combine chicken, fresh vegetables, salsa, and Monterey Jack cheese. No browning is involved. You can make this casserole for dinner and, if you're lucky, have leftovers for lunch the next day.

Prep Time: 15 minutes + baking
Oven Temperature: 350 degrees
Servings: 6 to 8

Ingredients

1½ pounds chicken thighs, skinless
1 package (1 ounce) taco seasoning, 40% less sodium
1 zucchini, cut in half, and then into half-moons
1 cup frozen corn, thawed
1 green pepper, thinly sliced
Salt and pepper to taste
1 jar (15 ounces) chunky salsa
8 ounces Monterey Jack cheese, reduced fat, shredded

Method

1. Heat oven to 350 degrees.
2. Coat casserole dish with cooking spray.
3. Lay chicken thighs in dish. Sprinkle taco seasoning over chicken.
4. Layer zucchini, corn, and green pepper over chicken. Season with salt and pepper to taste.
5. Spoon salsa over chicken and cover casserole with foil.
6. Bake 1 hour.
7. Remove foil.
8. Sprinkle Monterey Jack cheese over casserole and return to oven for 20 minutes.

Caregiver Tips

A 7-ounce can of fire-roasted green chiles, well drained, may be added to the casserole.

CHICKEN PAILLARDS WITH ARTICHOKES, TOMATOES, AND CHEESE

Chicken paillards are a smart choice for caregivers. A paillard is a thin piece of poultry or meat, pounded thin, and cooked quickly. Two slices of chicken have about 15 milligrams of cholesterol, 7.1 grams of protein, and 0.2 grams of fat—numbers that make chicken a healthy choice.

Prep Time: 15 minutes + baking
Oven Temperature: 350 degrees
Servings: 4

Ingredients
14 ounces chicken breasts, boneless/skinless
2 roma tomatoes
1 can (14 ounces) artichokes, packed in water, drained
2 tablespoons fresh basil, cut into thin ribbons
2 tablespoons olive oil
Salt and pepper to taste
1 cup Mozzarella cheese, reduced fat, shredded

Method

1. Heat oven to 350 degrees. Coat a baking dish with cooking spray.
2. Cut chicken breasts in half and place in plastic zipper bag. Seal bag and pound chicken with rolling pin until 1/4" thick.
3. Transfer chicken to dish.
4. Chop tomatoes and put in small bowl.
5. Chop artichokes and add to tomatoes.
6. Stir in basil, olive oil, salt, and pepper. Spoon over chicken.
7. Sprinkle cheese over all.
8. Cover with foil and bake at 350 degrees for 20 minutes.
9. Uncover and bake 10 more minutes, or until cheese starts to brown.

Caregiver Tips

Serve this with either microwavable rice, baked potatoes, or cooked orzo, and salad of your choice.

QUICK CHICK CASSEROLE

One day I looked in the refrigerator meat drawer and saw only one item: a package of cooked chicken strips from the deli. So it was chicken for dinner and this is the recipe I created. There are as many vegetables in this casserole as individual chicken pieces. This is fine with us, but you may wish to add more chicken.

Prep Time: 20 minutes + baking
Oven Temperature: 350 degrees
Servings: 4 to 5

Ingredients

2 cups noodles of your choice

2 tablespoons butter

1 box (8 ounces) button mushrooms, cleaned and sliced

1 can (10.5 ounces) cream of chicken soup, reduced sodium

1 soup can fat-free milk

1 teaspoon garlic powder

1½ cups sour cream, fat free

6 ounces chicken breast strips, oven roasted, from the deli or meat department

1 roasted red pepper from a jar, drained and chopped

2 tablespoons olive oil

1/2 cup Italian bread crumbs

Method

1. Heat oven to 350 degrees. Coat a baking dish with cooking spray.
2. Cook noodles al dente (not quite done) according to package directions. Rinse with cold water, drain, and transfer to bowl.
3. Melt butter in skillet. Add mushrooms and cook over medium heat until they start to brown. Remove from skillet and set aside.
4. Pour soup into skillet.
5. Add milk, garlic powder, and sour cream and warm over low heat.
6. Cut large chicken strips into smaller pieces.
7. Add chicken pieces, mushrooms, and red pepper to soup mixture. Transfer to baking dish.
8. Combine olive oil and bread crumbs and scatter over casserole. Cover with foil and bake ½ an hour.
9. Remove foil and bake 15 minutes more.

Caregiver Tips

You may add leftover vegetables, such as carrots or peas, to this recipe. Serve it for lunch or dinner.

CHICKEN, ZUCCHINI, AND ORZO

I love orzo (rice-shaped pasta) because it's such an adaptable ingredient. Orzo adds body and texture to soup, may be combined with peas for a side dish, served as the basis of a casserole, or become a main dish like this one. This recipe contains Herbes de Provence, a mixture of thyme, basil, savory, rosemary, fennel seeds, marjoram, and lavender flowers. Herbes de Provence made in France is costly. American manufacturers have a lower-priced version of this mixture, and one jar lasts a long time.

Prep Time: 25 minutes
Servings: 4

Ingredients

2 chicken bouillon cubes

1 cup orzo

2 tablespoons olive oil

2 chicken breasts, boneless/skinless, halved

1 teaspoon Herbes de Provence

Salt and pepper to taste

1 medium zucchini, shredded

1 lemon, zested and juiced
Cherry tomatoes, halved, for garnish

Method

1. Fill medium saucepan with water. Add bouillon cubes to water and cook orzo according to package directions.
2. Drain well, transfer to bowl, and cover with foil.
3. Pour olive oil into skillet.
4. Season chicken with Herbes de Provence, salt, and pepper.
5. Cook chicken on each side for 6 minutes.
6. Remove from skillet, put on plate, and cover with foil.
7. Add zucchini to skillet and cook over medium heat until crisp tender.
8. Combine zucchini and orzo.
9. Add lemon juice and zest to skillet.
10. Serve chicken over zucchini-orzo mixture, garnished with cherry tomatoes.

Caregiver Tips

You may add a chopped beefsteak tomato to the zucchini-orzo mixture.

CALIFORNIA-STYLE CHICKEN BURGERS WITH LETTUCE, TOMATO, AND AVOCADO

My sweet husband isn't a fan of chicken burgers, but he enjoyed this original recipe for them. Of course, he loves anything with avocado.

Prep Time: 25 minutes
Servings: 4

Ingredients

1 pound ground chicken breast

1 packet (1.5 ounces) taco seasoning, 40% less sodium

1 tablespoon olive oil

1/2 teaspoon salt

3 tablespoons red pepper, finely chopped

3 tablespoons green pepper, finely chopped

2 scallions, white and green parts, finely chopped

4 hamburger buns

Lettuce leaves, for garnish

1 beefsteak tomato, sliced, for garnish

1 avocado, sliced, for garnish

Method

1. Crumble chicken into bowl.
2. Add 1 tablespoon taco seasoning (save the rest), olive oil, salt, chopped peppers, and scallions.
3. Shape into four patties.
4. Coat skillet with cooking spray.
5. Cook burgers in skillet, turning when one side is brown.
6. Transfer to buns and top with lettuce, tomato, and avocado.

Caregiver Tips

You may enjoy a dollop of salsa on these burgers.

TURKEY, QUINOA, AND GRAPE SALAD

Quinoa is a protein-packed seed grown in the Andes Mountains. Peru is a main producer of quinoa. A friend of mine, another "foodie," and I were talking about trends, including quinoa. She gave me a pound of quinoa and told me how long to boil it. As the seeds swelled, the small dots in the middle of the seeds became visible. "When I looked into the pot I felt like hundreds of eyes were looking back at me," I told my friend. She couldn't stop laughing.

Prep Time: 15 minutes + boiling
Servings: 6

Ingredients

1 box (4.9 ounces) quinoa blend, your choice of flavor
1½ cups cooked turkey, cubed or shredded
2 scallions, white and green parts, chopped
1 cup green grapes, seedless, halved
1/3 cup dried cranberries
1/3 cup slaw dressing, light
2 tablespoons mayonnaise (reduced fat or fat free)

1 tablespoon honey
Lettuce leaves

Method

1. Cook quinoa according to package directions, about 15 minutes.
2. Remove cover and cool 10 minutes.
3. Add remaining ingredients (except lettuce) and combine well.
4. Spoon over lettuce leaves.

Caregiver Tips

You may eat this salad immediately or refrigerate for another time. Chopped Granny Smith apples may be substituted for grapes. Pair the salad with the popovers on page 215 and you have a delicious lunch or dinner.

HEALTHIER TURKEY TETRAZZINI

Wondering what to do with the last of the bird? This recipe may be the answer. I love turkey tetrazzini because my mother used to make it. I lightened the original recipe and here is the result.

Prep Time: 30 minutes + baking
Oven Temperature: 350 degrees
Servings: 12

Ingredients

1 box (16 ounces) spaghetti, extra fiber
4 tablespoons spreadable butter with canola oil + 1
    tablespoon butter for flavor
4 tablespoons flour, quick-mixing
2 cups fat-free milk
3 chicken bouillon cubes
1/8 teaspoon pepper
1 box (8 ounces) button mushrooms, cleaned and sliced
3 cups cooked turkey, cubed
1 package (10 ounces) cut asparagus, frozen (defrosted)
1 roasted red pepper from a jar, chopped
1½ cups Parmesan cheese, grated

Method

1. Break spaghetti in half and cook al dente according to package directions. Rinse with cold water, drain, and transfer to bowl.
2. Heat oven to 350 degrees.
3. Coat a 9" x 13" dish with cooking spray.
4. Melt spreadable butter in saucepan.
5. Whisk in flour, milk, bouillon cubes, and pepper. Cook over medium heat, stirring constantly, until sauce thickens.
6. Melt 1 tablespoon regular butter in skillet.
7. Cook mushrooms until they brown.
8. Add mushrooms, sauce, turkey, asparagus, and red pepper to cooked spaghetti.
9. Pour into baking dish. Sprinkle with Parmesan cheese.
10. Bake, uncovered, 30 minutes, or until sauce is bubbling and cheese is light brown.

Caregiver Tips

For a quicker version of this recipe make it with 1 can reduced-salt cream of mushroom soup, plus 3/4 soup can of milk. This casserole freezes well.

KENTUCKY HOT BROWN TURKEY SANDWICH

The classic Hot Brown Sandwich comes from the historic Brown Hotel in Louisville, Kentucky. It's an open-face turkey sandwich slathered with cheese sauce—a marvelous combination of flavors. The sauce is made with heavy cream, a caloric ingredient. To lighten the dish, I use fat-free milk, plain Romano cheese, and less turkey.

Prep Time: 20 minutes + broiling
Servings: 4

Ingredients

1½ tablespoons butter

1½ tablespoons flour, all-purpose or quick-mixing

1½ cups fat-free milk

1/4 cup Romano cheese, shredded, plus additional for garnish

Dash of nutmeg

Salt and pepper to taste

4 slices bread, toasted

1/2 pound (or more) turkey breast, sliced, available from the deli

2 roma tomatoes, quartered, for garnish
8 strips precooked bacon, for garnish

Method

1. Heat broiler.
2. Melt butter in saucepan over medium heat.
3. Whisk in flour and cook 1 minute.
4. Whisk in milk and cook over medium heat, stirring constantly, until sauce thickens. Remove from heat.
5. Add Romano cheese, nutmeg, salt, and pepper.
6. To assemble sandwiches, place 1 piece of toast in individual oven-safe dishes. Place several slices of turkey atop toast. Spoon some sauce over each sandwich.
7. Garnish with 2 pieces of tomato.
8. Sprinkle a little more cheese over sandwiches and broil until light brown.
9. Lay two pieces of bacon over each sandwich and serve.

Caregiver Tips

You may assemble this recipe like a casserole. Lay toast in the bottom of a shallow metal pan, put some sliced turkey on top of each one, 2 pieces of tomato by each piece of toast, and spoon sauce over all. Garnish with bacon just before serving.

STIR-FRIED TURKEY AND PEA PODS IN APRICOT SAUCE

Stir-fry is one of the quickest meals you can make. I keep a jar of apricot jam on hand just for this purpose. Peach jam works well too. The peach and apricot jams I use are the reduced-sugar variety.

Prep Time: 25 minutes
Servings: 2 to 3

Ingredients

2 tablespoons olive oil
1/2 pound turkey breast, cut into strips
1/2 yellow onion, halved and cut into crescents
1 cup pea pods, halved, strings removed
1 cup red pepper, cut into strips
1 teaspoon ginger paste
1/2 cup apricot jam, reduced sugar
2/3 cup chicken broth, reduced sodium
1–2 tablespoons cornstarch
1–2 tablespoons cold water
Cooked brown rice (or quinoa and brown rice blend)
Soy sauce, lower sodium, for garnish

Method

1. Pour 1 tablespoon olive oil in skillet.
2. Add turkey and cook over medium heat, stirring often.
3. Transfer turkey to plate.
4. Pour second tablespoon of oil into skillet.
5. Add onion, pea pods, red pepper, and ginger paste. Stir-fry for 2 minutes. Return turkey to skillet.
6. Add apricot jam and chicken broth.
7. Whisk water into cornstarch, making sure there are no lumps.
8. Slowly add mixture to skillet and cook over medium heat, stirring constantly, until sauce thickens.
9. Spoon over rice. Pass soy sauce if desired.

Caregiver Tips

For more apricot flavor, add some dried apricots that have been cut into thin strips.

COUNTRY CAPTAIN WITH GROUND CHICKEN OR TURKEY

Many cookbooks contain recipes for Country Captain. Popular as it is, nobody seems to know the origin of the recipe. I love this combination of savory and sweet flavors.

Prep Time: 20 minutes + simmering
Servings: 4 to 6

Ingredients

1/3 cup slivered almonds, toasted, for garnish
3 tablespoons olive oil
1 large yellow onion, chopped
1 green pepper, chopped
1 pound ground chicken or turkey
1 can (14.5 ounces) petite diced tomatoes in juice, no salt
1 tablespoon curry powder (more if you wish)
1 teaspoon salt (may be omitted)
1/2 teaspoon dried thyme
3 tablespoons tomato paste
1 teaspoon garlic powder
1/4 cup currants (or golden raisins)

1/2 cup water
Microwavable rice

Method

1. Toast almonds in dry skillet over low heat until they start to brown. Cool on plate.
2. Pour 1 tablespoon oil into skillet. Add onion and green pepper and cook until they start to brown. Remove and set aside.
3. Add second tablespoon of oil to skillet and cook poultry.
4. Return vegetables to skillet and add can of tomatoes, curry powder, salt, thyme, tomato paste, garlic powder, and currants.
5. Add water to skillet. Cover and cook 10 minutes.
6. Serve over rice and garnish with toasted almonds.

Caregiver Tips

Using ground poultry saves lots of time. Chop the onion and green pepper beforehand to save even more time.

Chapter 7

VEGETABLE RAINBOW

Steak House
Carrots and Onions
Page 152

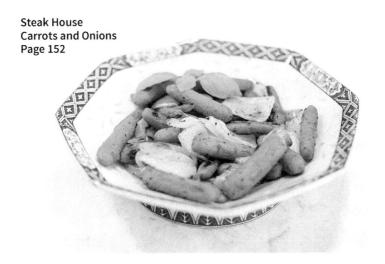

Vegetables contain vitamins, antioxidants, minerals, fiber, and other beneficial things. The US Government says your needed consumption of vegetables depends on age, gender, and amount of physical activity. Mayo Clinic, in its book, *Healthy Weight for Every Body*, says "fresh vegetables and fruits are the foundation of a healthy diet." One cup of raw vegetables is a serving. Two cups of raw, leafy vegetables is also a serving. Try a new vegetable today!

STEAK HOUSE CARROTS AND ONIONS

John and I went to a San Francisco steak house for dinner. The restaurant served only one vegetable—a combination of roasted carrots and onions—and I ordered them. When I tasted the vegetables I nearly swooned because they were so good. Since then, I've learned how to roast vegetables, and often use this cooking method. My family loves this steak house combo so much that I double the recipe.

Prep Time: 10 minutes + roasting
Oven Temperature: 425 degrees
Servings: 6

Ingredients
2 packages (1 pound each) carrots, petite or baby
2 large yellow onions, cut into chunks
3 tablespoons olive oil
1 tablespoon dried thyme
Salt and pepper to taste

Method

1. Heat oven to 425 degrees. Coat jelly roll pan with cooking spray.
2. Scatter carrots and onions on pan. Drizzle with olive oil, season with thyme, salt, and pepper, and toss to distribute seasonings.
3. Roast for 30–40 minutes, stirring several times, until the onions start to brown.

Caregiver Tips

You may also roast baby potatoes with the carrots and onions. Cut the potatoes in half, or into thirds.

THELMA'S ROLLED MUSHROOM SANDWICHES

I've belonged to The Study Club for decades. It's an historic club and the first reference to it appeared in an 1896 Rochester, Minnesota newspaper. Thelma was a member of the Club and when we met at her home, she always served mushroom sandwiches. They were yummy and I asked Thelma if she would share the recipe. She didn't. Years later, I received this letter from her:

Dear Harriet,
I found my recipe for rolled mushroom sandwiches at the bottom of a stack of unanswered mail—I cleaned my desk! Mea culpa. I really wanted you to have this recipe.

Thelma

Note: I changed Thelma's recipe a bit to suit a caregiver's schedule and needs.

Prep Time: 25 minutes + baking
Oven Temperature: 400 degrees
Baking Time: 10–12 minutes
Servings: 6

Ingredients

2 tablespoons butter

2 tablespoons minced onion (or scallions, white part only)

1 box (8 ounces) mushrooms, cleaned and sliced, finely chopped

1 clove garlic, minced or crushed in press

1/4 teaspoon nutmeg

3 tablespoons flour, all-purpose or quick-mixing

1 cup fat-free milk

6 slices bread, very fresh

Melted butter, for brushing sandwiches before heating

Method

1. Heat oven to 400 degrees.
2. Melt butter in a small saucepan.
3. Add onion and cook until soft.
4. Add mushrooms and sauté for 2 minutes.
5. Add garlic and nutmeg.
6. Sprinkle flour over mixture and stir in milk with wooden spoon. Cook over medium heat, stirring constantly, until thick. Cool sauce for 10 minutes.
7. Cut crusts off bread.

8. Put an equal amount of sauce on each sandwich and spread.
9. Roll sandwiches and place in shallow pan, seam side down.
10. Brush tops with melted butter and heat in oven until they start to brown.

Caregiver Tips

For extra color, add 1 tablespoon chopped parsley to the mushroom mixture. For extra flavor, sprinkle sandwiches with shredded Mozzarella cheese before rolling.

FRESH TOMATO SAUCE FOR PASTA

This is as fresh as pasta sauce gets and the basil adds a flavor punch. Use this recipe with all types of pasta. When I eat this sauce, I can almost smell tomatoes growing in the field.

Prep Time: About 15 minutes
Servings: 8

Ingredients

4 cups roma tomatoes, chopped
1 teaspoon garlic powder
1/2 cup fresh basil leaves, cut into ribbons
1/2 cup olive oil (or 2 tablespoons pasta water)
1 tablespoon red wine vinegar
Salt and pepper to taste
Hot pasta

Method

1. Combine all ingredients in medium bowl.
2. Toss with hot pasta.

Caregiver Tips

Some people seed the tomatoes before chopping them, but I don't, because I've learned that seeds contain vitamins. You may make this sauce with red and orange cherry tomatoes, cut into quarters.

BAKED TOMATOES CROWNED WITH SPINACH

This dish is a tasty "side" for hamburgers, steak, chicken, pork, or fish. It takes minutes to assemble—a plus for a busy caregiver like you. Besides, it's colorful and delicioius.

Prep Time: 20 minutes + baking
Oven Temperature: 350 degrees
Servings: 8

Ingredients

2–3 large beefsteak tomatoes, cut into thick slices

3 large eggs, beaten (or 3/4 cup egg substitute)

2 scallions, white and green parts, chopped

2 tablespoons olive oil (or butter, melted)

1/2 cup Mozzarella cheese, part skim, shredded

1/4 teaspoon garlic salt

1/4 teaspoon dried thyme

1 package (10 ounces) frozen chopped spinach, defrosted and drained

1 tablespoon butter, melted

3 tablespoons Italian bread crumbs (or Panko crumbs)

Method

1. Heat oven to 350 degrees. Coat a 9" x 13" dish with cooking spray.
2. Place tomato slices in baking dish.
3. Beat eggs, scallions, olive oil, Mozzarella, and seasonings together with fork.
4. Stir in spinach.
5. Spoon some spinach mixture on top of each tomato slice.
6. Combine melted butter and bread crumbs and sprinkle over tomatoes.
7. Bake, uncovered, for 20 minutes, or until cheese starts to brown.

Caregiver Tips

Cooked, shredded zucchini may be substituted for the spinach.

ARTICHOKE, MUSHROOM, AND RED PEPPER CASSEROLE

This vegetable combination is so yummy I could eat the entire casserole. I don't. Instead, I savor every spoonful of veggies, Parmesan cheese, and buttery bread crumbs. Ahhhh.

Prep Time: 25 minutes + baking
Oven Temperature: 325 degrees
Servings: 6

Ingredients

3 tablespoons olive oil
1 box (8 ounces) mushrooms, prewashed and sliced
3 scallions, white and green parts, chopped
1/4 cup roasted red pepper from a jar, drained and chopped
1 can (14 ounces) quartered artichokes, water packed, drained
2 tablespoons regular butter, for main recipe
2 tablespoons spreadable butter (or margarine), for main recipe
2 tablespoons flour (all-purpose or quick-mixing)

1/4 cup fat-free milk

3/4 cup water

1 teaspoon chicken base, reduced sodium (moist
    bouillon)

1/4 teaspoon dried thyme

3 tablespoons + 1/3 cup Parmesan cheese, grated

2 tablespoons butter, melted, for crumb topping

3 tablespoons Panko bread crumbs

Method

1. Heat oven to 325 degrees. Coat an 8" x 8" square
    baking dish with cooking spray.

2. Pour olive oil into large skillet. Cook mushrooms
    and scallions over medium heat until mushrooms are
    brown.

3. Remove skillet from heat and stir in chopped red
    pepper and artichokes.

4. Melt regular and spreadable butter in medium
    saucepan. Add flour and cook 1 minute.

5. Whisk in milk, water, chicken base, thyme, and 3
    tablespoons Parmesan cheese.

6. Cook over medium heat, stirring constantly, until
    sauce thickens.

7. Stir sauce into vegetables. Spoon mixture into
    prepared baking dish.

8. Put 2 tablespoons butter in microwavable measuring cup. Cover with plastic wrap and heat 20 seconds.
9. Stir butter into Panko bread crumbs and 1/3 cup Parmesan cheese. Scatter crumbs over casserole.
10. Bake 30 minutes or until edges start to bubble and topping starts to brown.

Caregiver Tips

Frozen artichokes, cooked and quartered, may be substituted for canned. However, this is a seasonal product and you may not be able to find it. Make this dish a few hours ahead of time, and bake it at the last minute. Save time by cooking the mushrooms a day ahead.

EASIEST MASHED POTATOES EVER

Shocking news: You make this recipe with instant mashed potatoes. I've served it to company many times and nobody, not one person, guessed the potatoes were instant. Many guests had second helpings. This casserole tastes good with almost any protein—steak, hamburgers, chicken, pork, and fish.

Prep Time: 15 minutes + baking
Oven Temperature: 350 degrees
Servings: 6

Ingredients

4 cups instant mashed potatoes
1 large egg, beaten
1 package (8 ounces) Neufchatel cheese, softened
1/2 teaspoon garlic powder
1 can (2.9 ounces) French-fried onions, for garnish

Method

1. Heat oven to 350 degrees. Coat a 1-quart casserole dish with cooking spray.
2. Hydrate potatoes according to package directions.
3. Add egg, neufchatel cheese, and garlic powder.
4. Transfer potatoes to casserole and top with French-fried onions.
5. Bake 30 minutes, covered, and 15 more minutes uncovered.

Caregiver Tips

For added flavor, butter the casserole dish and coat with Italian bread crumbs. Omit the onions and scatter a few more crumbs on top.

RED PEPPER DIP FOR VEGGIES

If your loved one doesn't like vegetables, this dip may spark her or his interest in them. The dip comes together in minutes and doesn't mask the flavor of the veggies.

Prep Time: 15 minutes + chilling
Servings: 6
Yield: 1½ cups

Ingredients

1 jar (8 ounces) roasted red peppers, drained
1 scallion, white and green parts, minced
1/2 cup mayonnaise, light
1/2 cup sour cream, fat free (or plain yogurt)
1/4 teaspoon garlic powder
Dash black pepper
Dash hot sauce
Bite-sized, raw vegetables to serve with dip: green pepper slices, broccoli florets, cauliflower florets, radishes, celery, carrots, cucumber slices

Method

1. Drain red peppers, dry with paper towels, and cut into chunks. Pureé in food processor or with a hand blender.
2. Add remaining ingredients.
3. Chill for 45 minutes to blend flavors.
4. Serve with a variety of raw vegetables.

Caregiver Tips

This dip tastes great with jicama, a root vegetable that tastes like an apple.

ROASTED ASPARAGUS BACON BUNDLES

Roasting asparagus is a new trend in my hometown. Although my husband isn't an asparagus fan, he is a bacon fan, and enjoys this recipe.

Prep Time: 20 minutes + roasting
Oven Time: 400 degrees
Servings: 5 to 6

Ingredients

1 bunch asparagus, woody ends removed
1 pound bacon
Cooking spray to coat tips and ends of finished bundles
Freshly ground black pepper

Method

1. Heat oven to 400 degrees. Cover bottom of a broiler pan with foil and coat top of pan with cooking spray.
2. Rinse asparagus under cold water and pat dry with paper towels.

3. Peel ends of spears. Wrap 3 or 4 together with bacon.

4. Set bundles on prepared pan, with loose bacon on the bottom.

5. Coat both ends of bundles with cooking spray and season asparagus with pepper.

6. Set pan on middle oven rack. Roast asparagus for about 15 minutes, turning once, until bacon is done.

7. If bacon isn't done, move pan to the top shelf and broil for a minute or so.

Caregiver Tips

Buy thin asparagus for easy preparation. If asparagus is fat, blanch in boiling water for 1½ minutes and cool enough to handle before wrapping with bacon. You may also roast plain asparagus for vegetarians.

GREEK VEGETABLE SKEWERS

When you are grilling skewers, it's a good idea to have separate skewers for vegetables and protein. These skewers taste best when charcoal grilled, but may be broiled in the oven.

Prep Time: 20 minutes + marinating and grilling
Servings: 8

Ingredients

1 large zucchini
1 yellow squash
2 red onions
1 red pepper
1 green pepper
8 fresh mushrooms
2 tablespoons lemon juice
2 tablespoons olive oil
1 teaspoon garlic salt
1 tablespoon dried rosemary

Method

1. Cut zucchini and yellow squash in half horizontally. Cut these sections into 1-inch pieces.
2. Cut the onions in half and again into chunks.
3. Seed peppers and cut into 1-inch pieces.
4. Clean mushrooms with paper towel.
5. Whisk lemon juice, olive oil, garlic salt, and rosemary together.
6. Thread vegetables onto metal skewers and lay in dish.
7. Pour lemon-oil mixture over them and marinate 1 hour.
8. Grill over medium-hot fire for 10–12 minutes, turning several times, until the vegetables start to char.

Caregiver Tips

Small eggplant may be substituted for other vegetables. Marinate the vegetables in bottled Greek dressing if you're pressed for time.

PASTA PRIMAVERA WITH OLIVE TAPENADE

Pasta and vegetables are a delicious, colorful, and satisfying meal. I've made many variations of this recipe and really like this one.

Prep Time: 30 minutes
Servings: 4 to 6

Ingredients

1 pound spaghetti, extra fiber
1 cup pasta water
2 tablespoons olive oil, divided
2 cloves garlic, minced (or 1 teaspoon garlic powder)
1 yellow onion, cut into chunks
1 box (8 ounces) button mushrooms, cleaned and sliced
1 zucchini, cut into thin, 2-inch sticks
2 cups cherry tomatoes, halved
1/4 cup green olive tapenade (or more)
About 6 fresh basil leaves, cut into thin strips with
    kitchen scissors, for garnish
Shredded Parmesan cheese, for garnish

Method

1. Cook pasta according to package directions. Reserve 1 cup pasta water.
2. Rinse pasta with cold water, drain, and set aside.
3. Pour 1 tablespoon olive oil into skillet and sauté garlic over medium heat until soft.
4. Add onion and cook until it starts to brown.
5. Pour second tablespoon of olive oil into same skillet and cook mushrooms until they start to brown.
6. Add zucchini. Cook a few more minutes until zucchini is crisp tender.
7. Add spaghetti, tomatoes, olive tapenade, and pasta water to skillet.
8. Cover and cook over low heat for 5 minutes.
9. Garnish with basil and Parmesan cheese.

Caregiver Tips

Green olive tapenade makes this pasta dish different. If you don't like olives, add 2 tablespoons small capers, drained.

ORANGE-GLAZED CARROTS

Carrots are naturally sweet. Adding marmalade and orange juice makes the carrots sweet *and* tangy. The cooking time depends on the type of marmalade you buy, one with only a little rind, or one with lots of rind. You may use low-sugar marmalade for this recipe.

Prep Time: 25 minutes
Servings: 8

Ingredients

2 packages (1 pound each) carrots, petite or baby, halved
2 tablespoons water
3/4 cup marmalade (regular, or reduced sugar)
1/4 cup orange juice
Dash of salt
Dash of pepper
Fresh Italian parsley, chopped, for garnish

Method

1. Dump carrots into microwavable dish. Add 2 tablespoons water, cover, and cook on high until tender, about 8 minutes.
2. Drain carrots.
3. Add remaining ingredients (except parsley) to dish. Cover and microwave 5–8 minutes.
4. Remove from microwave and stir to distribute sauce.
5. Garnish with chopped parsley.

Caregiver Tips

This recipe tastes especially good with pork or poultry.

CHEESY SPINACH-STUFFED BAKED POTATOES

Adults like stuffed potatoes (formerly called twice baked) and grandkids usually like them too. Bake the potatoes a day before you need them.

Prep Time: 15 minutes + baking
Oven temperature: 400 degrees
Servings: 4

Ingredients

2 large potatoes, baked
2 tablespoons butter (or spreadable butter with canola oil)
2/3 cup fat-free milk
1½ cups Mexican blend cheese, reduced fat, shredded
1/2 teaspoon salt (may be omitted)
Black pepper to taste
Half package (10 ounces in full package) frozen chopped spinach, defrosted and drained
1 package (2.5 ounces) real bacon pieces, for garnish

Method

1. Heat oven to 400 degrees.
2. Cut baked potatoes in half horizontally. With grapefruit knife, cut around rim of each potato half, being careful not to cut through bottom of shell.
3. Scoop out the flesh and transfer to large plate.
4. Mash potatoes with fork.
5. Set potato shells on rimmed pan.
6. Melt butter, milk, and 1 cup cheese in medium saucepan.
7. Add mashed potatoes and season with salt and pepper.
8. Stir in spinach and save the rest for another time.
9. Spoon mixture into shells and garnish with bacon pieces.
10. Bake for 15 minutes.

Caregiver Tips

Stuffed baked potatoes can be a vegetarian main dish. Cheddar or Pepper Jack cheese may be substituted for the Mexican blend. You may garnish the potatoes with French-fried onions instead of bacon.

Chapter 8

FABULOUS FRUITS

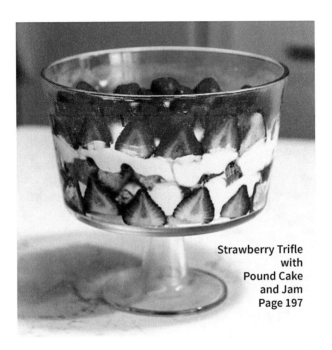

Strawberry Trifle
with
Pound Cake
and Jam
Page 197

When it comes to versatility, fruit gets the prize. You can eat it plain, combine it with other fruits, add it to main dishes, toss it in salads, stuff meat and poultry with it, use it in dessert recipes, dry it for later use, make special drinks with it, or turn it into jams and jellies. Fruit deserves another prize for health benefits because it's packed with vitamins. The recipes in this chapter use fruit in traditional and different ways. Fresh apples and pork are an historic combination. Adding fresh Mandarin orange segments to stir-fry is a different way to use fruit. To add more fruit to your diet, eat two fruits for breakfast.

FRAGRANT APPLE-CINNAMON GALETTE

Galette, (a one-crust pie with fruit in the center and a folded rim), takes less time to make than a two-crust pie. Once you've learned how to pleat the crust, the process goes quickly. You can't beat this combination of apples, sugar, and cinnamon warm from the oven.

Prep Time: 30 minutes + baking
Oven Temperature: 425 degrees
Servings: 6

Ingredients

1 refrigerated pie crust
3 cups apples, sliced
1/2 cup granulated sugar
2 tablespoons cornstarch
1 tablespoon lemon zest
1 tablespoon lemon juice
1/2 teaspoon cinnamon
2 tablespoons cold butter, cut into small pieces
2 tablespoons half and half

Extra granulated sugar, for top of galette
Whipped cream or frozen vanilla yogurt, for garnish

Method

1. Heat oven to 425 degrees.
2. Cover the bottom of a jelly roll pan with parchment paper and set crust on parchment.
3. In a large bowl, combine apples, sugar, cornstarch, lemon zest, lemon juice, and cinnamon.
4. Spoon mixture in center of crust, leaving a 1/2-inch margin around edge.
5. Fold edge of dough in one direction. Leave 1½ inches, and fold again. Continue pleating as you go.
6. Dot the top of galette with cold butter.
7. Brush pleated rim with half and half and sprinkle with granulated sugar.
8. Bake pie 25–30 minutes, or until edges start to brown.
9. Cool 1/2 hour and cut into slices.
10. Top each serving with whipped cream or frozen yogurt.

Caregiver Tips

Slicing the apples with a box grater saves even more time. You may add 1/2 cup currants to the apples for color and flavor. This recipe works with peaches, strawberries, blueberries, blackberries, or a combination of berries.

BRITTANY PORK CHOPS WITH BACON, APPLES, AND ONIONS

The apples add sweetness and moisture to this recipe. Serve with ready-made, refrigerated mashed potatoes or microwavable rice.

Prep Time: 25 minutes + baking
Oven Temperature: 375 degrees
Servings: 4

Ingredients

4 center-cut pork chops, boneless
1 large onion, peeled, thinly sliced
1–2 tablespoons butter
8 slices precooked bacon, crumbled
2 Granny Smith apples, peeled and sliced
1/3 cup dried cranberries, with 50% less sugar
1/2 cup white wine (or apple juice)
Parsley (optional), for garnish

Method

1. Coat a casserole dish and skillet with cooking spray. Set dish aside.
2. Place pork chops in skillet and brown both sides.
3. Transfer chops to casserole dish.
4. Scatter some onion slices on top of each chop.
5. Dot with butter.
6. Crumble bacon over chops.
7. Top with sliced apples and dried cranberries.
8. Add wine (or juice), cover, and bake at 375 degrees for 1 hour.
9. Garnish with parsley if desired.

Caregiver Tips

If you double or triple this recipe, bake chops in a Dutch oven. Layer the ingredients: chops, onions, butter, bacon, and cranberries. I like the sauce just the way it is, but you may wish to thicken it with a little cornstarch dissolved in cold water.

PEARS DRENCHED IN RED WINE

I love these pears and really love the syrup, which is why I make double the amount. This dessert may be served warm or cold.

Prep Time: 20 minutes + simmering and cooling
Servings: 6

Ingredients

6 pears, soft but not mushy
2 lemons, washed
4 cups red wine (burgundy, cabernet, or merlot)
2 cups granulated sugar
4 tablespoons raspberry jam, sugar free

Method

1. Peel pears and remove cores with potato peeler or paring knife.
2. Cut a small slice from the bottom of each pear so it can stand upright.

3. Remove some rind from each lemon and slice into thin strips.
4. Squeeze lemons and set juice aside.
5. In a large saucepan, combine lemon rind, wine, and sugar. Simmer over medium heat, uncovered, for 5 minutes.
6. Set pears in syrup. Cover and simmer on low heat for 35 minutes, or until a sharp knife goes into pears easily.
7. Using a slotted spoon, remove pears from syrup, and place in individual serving dishes.
8. Stir lemon juice and raspberry jam into warm syrup.
9. Spoon some over each pear and cool pears on counter for 1/2 hour.
10. Serve warm.

Caregiver Tips

You may garnish each serving with mint, lemon zest, or shaved chocolate.

SCANDINAVIAN FRUIT "SOUP"

The idea of a cold fruit soup comes from Sweden. This so-called soup is really a thin pudding with added fruit. You may serve this recipe as an appetizer or dessert.

Prep Time: 30 minutes + chilling
Servings: 12

Ingredients

4 cups orange juice
1 cup water
3/4 cup granulated sugar
3 whole cloves
1 cinnamon stick
6 tablespoons cornstarch
1 cup water
1 cup strawberries, sliced
1 cup seedless green grapes, halved
2 oranges, peeled and sectioned or 1 cup Mandarin
    oranges, drained
Mint leaves (optional), for garnish

Method

1. Combine orange juice, water, sugar, cloves, and cinnamon stick in medium saucepan.
2. Cook over medium heat until sugar dissolves, about 10 minutes.
3. While mixture is heating, whisk cornstarch and water together, making sure there are no lumps.
4. Drizzle cornstarch mixture into syrup, stirring constantly, and cook until pudding is thick and clear.
5. Transfer to large bowl. Cover and chill for at least 1–2 hours.
6. Remove cloves and cinnamon stick.
7. Gently stir fruit into pudding and garnish with mint if desired.

Caregiver Tips

Other fresh fruit—blueberries, raspberries, melon balls, red grapes, and so on—may be added to the "soup."

CRUNCHY PEAR AND CHICKEN SALAD

Fruit livens up meats and salads. This salad, made with pears, dried cranberries, baby spinach, and chicken, can be a lunch or dinner.

Prep Time: 25 minutes
Servings: 4

Ingredients
2 cups rotisserie chicken, shredded
1 large rib celery, chopped
2 tablespoons red onion, finely chopped
2 fresh pears, seeded and thinly sliced
1/4 cup dried cranberries, with 50% less sugar
Light slaw dressing
Chow mein noodles, for garnish
Prewashed baby spinach

Method

1. Combine all ingredients, except slaw dressing, chow mein noodles, and spinach, in a large bowl.
2. Drizzle slaw dressing over salad and toss gently.
3. Place some baby spinach on individual plates. Spoon salad over spinach.
4. Garnish with chow mein noodles.

Caregiver Tips

Chopped dried apricots may be substituted for the cranberries. This salad goes nicely with the giant popovers on page 215.

RED AND GREEN GRAPES IN SOUR CREAM SAUCE

This simple recipe is just plain delicious—a light ending to any meal. Some people are allergic to walnuts and if you're one of them, use sliced almonds instead.

Prep Time: 15 minutes + chilling
Servings: 4 to 5

Ingredients

1/2 cup walnut pieces
3 tablespoons dark brown sugar
1 teaspoon pure vanilla extract
Dash of nutmeg
1 cup sour cream, fat free
1 cup seedless green grapes, halved
1 cup seedless red grapes, halved

Method

1. Toast walnuts in dry skillet over low heat until they start to brown. Cool on plate.
2. Stir sugar, vanilla extract, and nutmeg into sour cream.
3. Add grapes and walnuts.
4. Refrigerate for 1/2 hour.
5. Spoon into individual serving dishes.

Caregiver Tips

If you make this dessert too far ahead, the grape juice dilutes the sauce. To prevent this from happening, keep the fruit and sauce separate until serving.

MANDARIN ORANGE ALMOND CHICKEN

You'll like this recipe if you like the pairing of orange and chicken. This recipe has fewer calories than the restaurant version because the chicken isn't battered or fried; it's stir-fried. Almonds give this dish extra crunch.

Prep Time: 30 minutes
Servings: 6 to 8

Ingredients

1/3 cup sliced almonds, for garnish
1 Mandarin orange, peeled and segmented, for garnish
   (both orange and peel)
1 package (14 ounces) chicken tenders
2 tablespoons olive oil
3 scallions, washed and sliced into 1-inch diagonal pieces
1 cup orange juice
1/2 cup chicken broth, no salt
1 tablespoon honey
1/2 teaspoon garlic powder
1/8 teaspoon crushed red pepper flakes
1 tablespoon soy sauce, reduced sodium

1 tablespoon water
1½ tablespoons cornstarch
1 package (8 ounces) microwavable brown rice

Method

1. Toast almonds in dry skillet over medium heat. Cool on plate.
2. Cut peel off orange and save half.
3. Slice peel into thin strips and cut these strips in half. Set aside.
4. Cut chicken into 1-inch pieces.
5. Pour olive oil into skillet and heat until hot.
6. Stir-fry chicken and cook until it starts to brown.
7. Add scallions, orange juice, chicken broth, honey, garlic powder, red pepper flakes, and soy sauce. Cover and simmer 5 minutes.
8. Whisk water into cornstarch, making sure there are no lumps. Drizzle into skillet mixture and cook over medium heat, stirring constantly, until sauce thickens.
9. Cook rice 90 seconds, according to package instructions.
10. Spoon chicken mixture over rice, and garnish with orange segments and almonds.

Caregiver Tips

For a more complete meal, add 1/3 cup frozen peas to skillet. This dish tastes good with frozen egg rolls, cooked as directed.

STRAWBERRY TRIFLE WITH POUND CAKE AND JAM

British Trifle, a dessert made with sherry-soaked cake, custard, jam, and whipped cream, goes back hundreds of years. Because of the sherry, the dessert was known as Tipsy Hedgehog, Tipsy Squire, Tipsy Pudding, Tipsy Parson, and Tipsy Cake, according to the Decadent Desserts website. Some believe the dessert originated as a way to use up stale cake. Presentation is key to the success of this dessert and you need a trifle bowl. My recipe doesn't contain sherry, so kids can eat it. People will gasp when you bring out this festive dessert.

Prep Time: 20 minutes + chilling
Servings: 8

Ingredients

1 cup sliced almonds, toasted, for garnish

1½ cups skim milk

1 teaspoon pure almond extract

1 box (1 ounce) instant vanilla pudding mix (regular or sugar free)

1 carton (8 ounces) whipped topping, sugar free, or 2
   cups whipped cream
1 pound cake, frozen (plain or blueberry)
1 pint fresh strawberries, halved, for layering
Sugar-free strawberry jam, for layering and garnish
Whipped cream, for garnish (may be omitted)

Method

1. Toast almonds in a dry skillet over low heat until they
   start to brown. Cool on plate.
2. Whisk milk and almond extract into pudding mix and
   refrigerate 1 hour.
3. Fold whipped topping into pudding.
4. Slice pound cake in half horizontally, and cut into
   1-inch cubes.
5. Put a layer of cake cubes on the bottom of trifle bowl.
   Sprinkle with a few strawberries.
6. Spread jam over berries and add a layer of pudding.
7. Continue layering until ingredients are gone.
8. Top trifle with whipped cream and garnish with
   toasted almonds.

Caregiver Tips

Depending on price, you may wish to add another pint of strawberries. You can also make an all-peach trifle with peach jam. Chocolate angel food cake and raspberries are another winning combination. This recipe tastes best with real whipped cream.

FRESH FRUIT COMPOTE

Fruit can be a refreshing side dish or sweet dessert. This combination of fruits is both. Serve it plain as a side for spaghetti, lasagna, or barbecue. Add some white wine or sauterne for a sweet ending to any meal.

Prep Time: 25 minutes + chilling
Servings: 12

Ingredients

2 ripe nectarines
1 cup seedless green grapes, halved
1 cup seedless red grapes, halved
2 tangerines, peeled and sectioned
1 medium cantaloupe, cubed
1 banana, sliced
1/3 cup orange juice
2 cups white wine (or juice of your choice), for garnish

Method

1. Wash fruit.
2. Cut nectarines into slices. Place in large bowl.
3. Add grapes, tangerines, cantaloupe, and banana.
4. Pour orange juice over fruit and combine gently.
5. Serve immediately or chill 1 hour.
6. For dessert, add wine to fruit mélange just before serving.

Caregiver Tips

Fresh fruit can be a welcome contrast to a spicy meal. This compote will help your loved one get the recommended number of fruits and vegetables a day.

APRICOT AND ALMOND RICE

Searching for a rice dish that goes with everything? This is the one. White or brown rice is simmered in chicken broth with dried apricots. When the rice is done, it's garnished with toasted almonds. This rice tastes good with beef, chicken, pork, or fish.

Prep Time: 20 minutes
Servings: 6
Yield: 3 cups

Ingredients

1 tablespoon olive oil
1 teaspoon butter
1 medium yellow onion, chopped
1 cup brown rice, uncooked
1¾ cups chicken broth, no salt
1/2 cup dried apricots, cut into small strips
1/2 cup golden raisins
3/4 cup slivered almonds, toasted, for garnish

Method

1. Put olive oil and butter in large saucepan.
2. As soon as the butter has melted, add onion and cook until it starts to brown.
3. Add rice, chicken broth, apricots, and raisins.
4. Cover and cook rice according to instructions on brown rice bag.
5. While rice is cooking, sauté almonds in dry skillet until they start to brown. Cool on plate.
6. Garnish cooked rice with toasted almonds.

Caregiver Tips

Make this recipe ahead of time and heat in the microwave later. Add a couple tablespoons of water if the rice seems dry, cover with plastic wrap, and heat on high for 2 minutes.

Chapter 9

MUFFINS AND BREADS

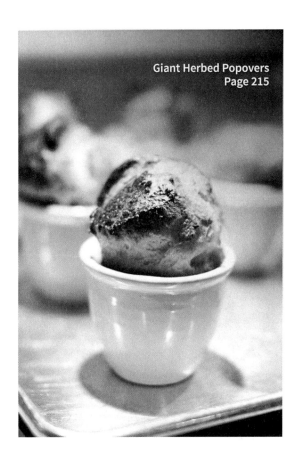

Giant Herbed Popovers
Page 215

Baking is a satisfying experience. The house smells wonderful and your efforts are rewarded. I'm reluctant to admit it, but I rarely make a recipe as written, and usually alter it to suit my tastes. Baking is the exception to this, and the ingredients must be measured accurately. No cheating! Spooning flour into a measuring cup and leveling it with a knife is more accurate than scooping flour, which compresses it. Densely packed flour can skew recipe results.

SURPRISE CORN MUFFINS

Corn muffins go with many foods—barbecued pork and beef, ham, chili, and casseroles. I think these muffins taste best at breakfast, but you can eat them anytime. As soon as you've eaten one, chances are you'll want another.

Prep Time: 15 minutes + baking
Oven Temperature: 400 degrees
Servings: 6

Ingredients

1/3 cup fat-free milk
2 tablespoons honey
1/2 teaspoon pure vanilla extract
1 large egg
1 package (8.5 ounces) corn muffin mix
6 teaspoons strawberry jam
Sugar, for sprinkling muffin tops (may be omitted)

Method

1. Heat oven to 400 degrees. Coat muffin pan with cooking spray.

2. Whisk milk, honey, vanilla, and egg together in batter bowl.
3. Stir in corn muffin mix.
4. Ladle into muffin cups and fill half-full.
5. Drop 1 teaspoon of jam on top of each muffin.
6. Cover with remaining batter.
7. Sprinkle tops with sugar.
8. Bake about 20 minutes, or until tops are golden brown.

Caregiver Tips

Until I became a family caregiver, I made corn muffins from scratch. Now I use a mix and the muffins still taste like they're made from scratch. Don't use strawberry spread for this recipe because it will sink to the bottom of the muffin pan.

CHOCOLATE DESSERT WAFFLES

Waffles can be transformed into a dessert buffet. Ask family members and friends to make their own waffles and choose their own toppings. Chocolate waffles are especially good with frozen yogurt and reduced-sugar or sugar-free chocolate sauce.

Prep Time: 10 minutes + baking
Servings: 3 whole waffles (12 dessert-sized)

Ingredients

1 cup baking mix, spooned and leveled
1 cup fat-free milk
1 egg, beaten
1/2 cup sweetened cocoa powder (4 packets)
1 tablespoon sugar
1 teaspoon pure vanilla extract
1 tablespoon olive oil (or melted butter)
Toppings: Strawberries, raspberries, canned cherries in syrup, whipped cream, vanilla ice cream, coffee ice cream, chocolate ice cream, chocolate sauce, and sprinkles

Method

1. Heat waffle maker.
2. Combine all ingredients in batter bowl.
3. Cook in waffle iron and serve immediately with choice of toppings.

Caregiver Tips

You may make the waffles ahead of time and freeze them. For more chocolate flavor add 1/2 cup mini chocolate chips to batter.

PUMPKIN AND SPICE PANCAKES

These fragrant pancakes are a wonderful breakfast. Serve them for supper with bacon, sausage, and fresh fruit cups—a mixture of seasonal fruits from the market.

Prep Time: 12 minutes + cooking
Skillet Temperature: 350 degrees
Servings: 8

Ingredients

1 cup baking mix, spooned and leveled
1 teaspoon ground cinnamon
1/2 teaspoon allspice
1 tablespoon sugar
1/2 cup canned pumpkin (save the rest)
1 large egg (or 2 tablespoons egg substitute)
1 cup fat-free milk
Maple syrup, reduced-sugar syrup (or sugar-free syrup)

Method

1. Whisk ingredients except syrup together in a large batter bowl.

2. Set nonstick electric skillet to 350 degrees or regular skillet to medium heat.
3. Cook pancakes on one side until top bubbles.
4. Flip pancakes and finish cooking.
5. Serve immediately with warm syrup, reduced-sugar syrup, or sugar-free syrup.

Caregiver Tips
Add a thinly sliced apple to the syrup for extra flavor.

GRANNY SMITH'S APPLE-DAPPLE MUFFINS

With applesauce and chopped apples, this recipe has a double burst of apple flavor. The paid caregivers who come for two hours each morning love these muffins.

Prep Time: 15 minutes + baking
Oven Temperature: 400 degrees
Servings: 12

Ingredients

1/2 cup applesauce, sugar free
1/2 cup granulated sugar
1/2 cup vegetable oil
2 large eggs, room temperature
1 teaspoon pure vanilla extract
2 cups all-purpose flour, spooned and leveled
3/4 teaspoon baking soda
3/4 teaspoon ground cinnamon
1/2 teaspoon salt
1½ cups Granny Smith apples (1 large), peeled and
    chopped

Method

1. Heat oven to 400 degrees. Coat 2 muffin pans with cooking spray.
2. In a batter bowl, whisk applesauce, sugar, vegetable oil, eggs, and vanilla together.
3. In another bowl, whisk dry ingredients together.
4. Slowly add dry ingredients to wet.
5. Fold in chopped apples.
6. Spoon into muffin tins and bake 25 minutes, or until muffins start to pull away from pan.
7. Remove muffins from oven.
8. Using a table knife, cut around each muffin and tilt sideways to cool.

Caregiver Tips

Grating the apple saves you a few minutes, but the apple will meld with the batter, and you won't bite into chunks.

GIANT HERBED POPOVERS

A friend of mine had a catering business, in addition to his regular job. Both of us were foodies and we talked about recipes whenever we met. I offered to share my popover recipe with him and said they would be six inches high. Weeks later I received a note from my friend, thanking me for the recipe, and correcting my height estimate. "The popovers weren't six inches high," he wrote. "They were seven inches high!"

Prep Time: 10 minutes + baking
Oven Temperature: 400 degrees
Servings: 6

Ingredients

3 large eggs, room temperature
1¼ cups fat-free milk
1 tablespoon olive oil (or canola)
1/2 teaspoon salt
1 teaspoon dried thyme
1¼ cups flour (all-purpose), spooned and leveled

Method

1. Heat oven to 400 degrees.
2. Liberally grease 6 custard cups with shortening. Set on jelly roll pan.
3. In a batter bowl, whisk eggs, milk, oil, salt, and thyme together.
4. Whisk in flour.
5. Ladle batter into cups and bake 30–35 minutes.

Caregiver Tips

The height of these popovers depends on the size and shape of the custard cups. I grease the cups with Crisco. For a flavor variation, add 1/4 cup grated Parmesan or Cheddar cheese to the batter.

MARMALADE MUFFINS WITH ORANGE DRIZZLE

I always have marmalade on the shelf and use it in a variety of ways. The marmalade in this recipe gives you the orange flavor without extra work—no peeling, segmenting, or squeezing oranges. Still, you smell oranges and taste their refreshing flavor.

Prep Time: 15 minutes + baking
Oven Temperature: 400 degrees
Servings: 12

Ingredients

2 cups all-purpose flour, spooned and leveled
1 teaspoon baking powder
1 teaspoon baking soda
1/2 teaspoon salt
1 carton (8 ounces) lemon yogurt (or plain)
2/3 cup marmalade (regular or reduced sugar)
1/4 cup butter, melted (or vegetable oil)
1 large egg, beaten
1½ teaspoons orange extract
1/2 teaspoon pure vanilla extract

3/4 cup powdered sugar, for frosting
1 tablespoon orange juice, for frosting

Method

1. Heat oven to 400 degrees. Coat 2 muffin pans with cooking spray.
2. In a batter bowl, whisk dry ingredients, except powdered sugar, together.
3. In another bowl, whisk yogurt, marmalade, butter, egg, and extracts together.
4. Add wet ingredients to dry, stirring just enough to combine.
5. Spoon batter into muffin pans and bake 25 minutes, or until toothpick comes out clean.
6. Remove muffins from oven and cool on wire rack for 10 minutes.
7. Set muffins on wax paper.
8. Stir orange juice into powdered sugar and drizzle frosting over muffin tops.

Caregiver Tips

Omit the glaze if you're pressed for time. Just sprinkle the muffins with sugar and bake them.

CHEESY BUTTERMILK DROP BISCUITS

Drop biscuits are quick to make and bake. Cheddar cheese and tangy buttermilk make these biscuits special. Although biscuit mixes are available, you're paying the manufacturer to measure, package, and market the ingredients—and you still have to add liquid and cheese. Homemade biscuits are much less expensive. These biscuits taste great with stew and, like all biscuits, taste best when warm.

Prep Time: 20 minutes + baking
Oven Temperature: 450 degrees
Servings: 14

Ingredients
2 cups all-purpose flour, spooned and leveled
2 teaspoons baking powder
1/4 teaspoon baking soda
1 teaspoon garlic powder
1 teaspoon salt
5 tablespoons cold butter, cut into small pieces
1 cup Cheddar cheese, reduced fat, shredded
1 cup buttermilk, reduced fat

Method

1. Heat oven to 450 degrees. Coat baking pan with cooking spray.
2. Whisk flour, baking powder, baking soda, garlic powder, and salt together.
3. Cut butter into flour with pastry blender until it resembles crumbs.
4. Stir shredded cheese into mixture.
5. Add buttermilk and combine well. (Make sure you incorporate all of the flour in the bottom of the bowl.)
6. Drop by tablespoonfuls onto prepared pan.
7. Bake 12–15 minutes or until golden.

Caregiver Tips

These biscuits brown quickly, so you need to watch them carefully, or they will burn. The biscuits may be brushed with melted butter before serving. Tempted as you may be, don't use powdered buttermilk for this recipe because the biscuits won't taste as good.

VERY BRITISH YORKSHIRE PUDDING

My mother's parents came to America from Sheffield, England and brought their love of Yorkshire pudding with them. Mom learned to make this recipe from her mother. I learned to make it from my mother. Although the original recipe uses meat fat to prevent the pudding from sticking to the pan, I use cooking spray. Roast beef was a special treat at our house and Mom always made extra gravy. When the meat was gone, we had Yorkshire pudding and gravy for dinner, sans meat. I loved it!

Prep Time: 10 minutes + baking
Oven Temperature: 450 degrees
Servings: 6

Ingredients

3 large eggs, room temperature
1 cup fat-free milk
3/4 teaspoon salt
1 cup all-purpose flour, spooned and leveled
Gravy (to serve alongside)

Method

1. Heat oven to 450 degrees. Coat a metal pie plate with cooking spray.
2. In a batter bowl, whisk eggs, milk, and salt together.
3. Whisk in flour and pour into prepared pan.
4. Bake 15 minutes.
5. Lower temperature to 350 degrees and bake 15 more minutes, until pudding is puffed and golden brown.
6. Serve immediately with gravy.

Caregiver Tips

I've used part eggs and part egg substitute for this recipe, but regular eggs work best.

PARMESAN TOASTS

I'm a little embarrassed to include this recipe, but friends have asked for it. "These are really good!" one exclaimed. "How do you make them?" Parmesan Toasts take only minutes to make, and go well with spaghetti, lasagna, salads, soups, and other meals.

Prep Time: 10 minutes + broiling
Broiler Temperature: 425 degrees
Servings: 4

Ingredients

4 slices bread
Butter (or herbed butter on page 79)
1 carton (8 ounces) Parmesan cheese, grated (or
    Parmesan and Romano)
Freshly ground black pepper

Method

1. Heat oven broiler.
2. Cut crusts off bread and spread each slice with plain or herbed butter.

3. Sprinkle with Parmesan cheese and a little pepper.
4. Cut each slice into three "fingers."
5. Set fingers on metal pan.
6. Broil 3 minutes, or until Parmesan cheese starts to brown. Serve warm.

Caregiver Tips

You may use wheat, sourdough, rye, olive, or other kinds of bread for this recipe. Make sure the grated cheese you buy doesn't contain any fillers because it doesn't take as good. Parmesan Toasts may also be cooked in a toaster oven.

Chapter 10

SWEET TOOTH

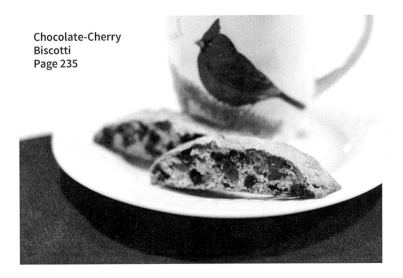

Chocolate-Cherry
Biscotti
Page 235

My mother was an excellent baker and used to bake desserts for church suppers. There were no mixes at the time, and every dessert was homemade: orange sponge cake, banana bread, and date-nut bread so rich it seemed like a dessert. One day she made a chocolate layer cake and left it on the kitchen table while she dressed for church. When she returned the plate was empty. Our cocker spaniel, Timmy, had eaten the whole thing! Timmy was so full he could hardly walk, yet he looked happy. You'll be happy after you taste these recipes.

FUDGY PUDDING

Pudding mixes are convenient, but I think homemade tastes better. I've made vanilla, butterscotch, cinnamon, and chocolate pudding from scratch and all were delicious. This recipe uses baking chocolate, which gives the pudding its fudgy flavor.

Prep Time: 15 minutes + chilling
Servings: 8

Ingredients

2½ squares chocolate, unsweetened

2 tablespoons + 1 tablespoon butter

3½ cups fat-free milk (or 2% or whole milk)

1/3 cup cornstarch

3/4 cup sugar

1/4 teaspoon salt

1 teaspoon pure vanilla extract

Whipped cream or whipped topping, sugar free, for garnish

Chocolate or colored sprinkles (optional), for garnish

Method

1. In small saucepan, melt chocolate and 2 tablespoons butter over low heat.
2. Warm milk in another pan.
3. Whisk cornstarch, sugar, and salt together.
4. Stir dry mixture into melted chocolate-butter mixture.
5. Slowly add this mixture to milk. Cook over medium heat, stirring several times, until pudding thickens. (The chocolate specks will slowly disappear.)
6. Remove pudding from heat. Add vanilla extract and last tablespoon of butter.
7. Spoon into serving dishes and chill 1 hour or more.
8. Top with whipped cream or topping and garnish with sprinkles.

Caregiver Tips

This pudding is firm enough for pie. For softer pudding, add another half cup of milk. Pudding is a good source of calcium for your loved one.

RASPBERRY PANNA COTTA

Panna Cotta is a flavorful ending to any meal. This dessert is also known as Swedish Cream, Russian Cream, and Italian Panna Cotta. I lightened the recipe by using fat-free evaporated milk and fat-free sour cream. I love almond, so I added pure almond extract to the recipe.

Prep Time: 15 minutes + chilling
Servings: 12

Ingredients

2 cups sugar
1/2 teaspoon salt
2 envelopes unflavored gelatin
2½ pints evaporated milk, fat free
3 cups sour cream, fat free
1 teaspoon pure vanilla extract
1½ teaspoons pure almond extract
1 box (8 ounces) raspberries, fresh, for garnish
Raspberry jam, sugar free, for garnish
Water, to thin out raspberry jam

Method

1. Combine sugar, salt, and gelatin in a large saucepan.
2. Gradually add evaporated milk.
3. Cook over low heat, stirring occasionally, until gelatin and sugar are dissolved and mixture coats a spoon. Do not allow mixture to boil.
4. Remove pan from heat. Stir in sour cream and extracts
5. Pour into bowl or individual serving dishes.
6. Cover and chill until completely set.
7. Top with fresh raspberries. Thin raspberry jam with a little water and drizzle over berries.

Caregiver Tips

Not only is this a delicious dessert, but you can make it hours ahead. Fresh peaches and peach jam may be substituted for raspberries.

ITALIAN BISCUIT TORTONI

I've made this fancy ice cream dessert from scratch, and it was time consuming. First, I made a custard base and chilled it. Next, I folded whipped cream into the base. Then I added crumbled macaroons, cherries, and almonds to this mixture, and froze it. You may save time by making this ice cream version of Biscuit Tortoni.

Prep Time: 25 minutes + freezing
Servings: 12

Ingredients
1 carton (1.5 quarts) vanilla ice cream or yogurt
1 cup crumbled macaroon cookies
1/2 cup Maraschino cherries, drained and halved
1/2 cup salted almonds, chopped

Method
1. Take ice cream out of freezer and microwave on high for 15 seconds. If it doesn't start to melt, microwave a few seconds more.

2. Remove ice cream from carton. Cut into sections with serrated knife.
3. Put sections into large bowl.
4. Working quickly, fold in crumbled cookies, cherries, and almonds.
5. Transfer to large storage container and refreeze.

Caregiver Tips

Thawing takes some of the air out of the ice cream, so it will be denser than usual. This is a rich dessert and you may wish to reduce the serving size. Individual servings may be frozen in paper cups.

HARRIET'S DOUBLE ALMOND COOKIES

Baking is satisfying, even therapeutic, and that's why I included this cookie recipe. My grandson loves these cookies so much he thought I should sell them at Rochester's summer festival. "You could sell them warm," he continued. I won't be selling cookies at the festival, but I'm glad to share my best cookie recipe with you. Make the dough a day ahead and refrigerate. Roll into balls and bake the next day.

Prep Time: 20 minutes + baking
Oven Temperature: 350 degrees
Yield: 5 dozen

Ingredients
1 cup butter (or butter-flavored Crisco)
1/3 cup dark brown sugar
1 cup granulated sugar, plus extra to roll dough in
2 large eggs, room temperature
1 tablespoon pure almond extract
1 teaspoon water

1½ cups all-purpose flour
1½ cups wheat flour
1/2 teaspoon salt
1 package (3.25 ounces) whole almonds, for garnish

Method

1. Heat oven to 350 degrees.
2. Cream butter, brown sugar, and granulated sugar together with electric mixer.
3. Add eggs, almond extract, and water.
4. Whisk dry ingredients, except almonds, together. Slowly add to creamed mixture, finishing with wooden spoon if necessary.
5. Form dough into small balls and roll in granulated sugar.
6. Set on baking sheet with 2 inches between cookies.
7. Flatten dough balls with a glass bottom dipped in sugar.
8. Put whole almond in the center of each cookie.
9. Bake 10 minutes, or just until edges start to brown. Don't over-bake.
10. Cool cookies for a few seconds before removing from pan.

Caregiver Tips

Admittedly, 5 dozen cookies is a lot, but you can freeze a few dozen. Although these aren't fortune cookies, every time I make them I think I'll have good fortune. Double Almond Cookies are always a welcome gift.

CHOCOLATE-CHERRY BISCOTTI

I love to make biscotti and often give it for gifts. Although many recipes require an electric mixer, I take the easy route and make biscotti with a whisk, wooden spoon, and batter bowl. Biscotti keeps for weeks when stored in an air-tight container.

Prep Time: 15 minutes + baking and cooling
Oven Temperature: 325 degrees
Yield: 3 dozen

Ingredients

2¼ cups all-purpose flour (or half-white and half-wheat)

1 teaspoon baking powder

1/2 teaspoon baking soda

1 cup mini chocolate chips (or sugar-free chocolate chips)

1 cup candied cherries, chopped

1 cup granulated sugar

2 large eggs, room temperature

1/2 cup egg substitute

2 teaspoons pure vanilla extract

Method

1. Heat oven to 325 degrees. Coat jelly roll pan with cooking spray.
2. In a large bowl, whisk together flour, baking powder, baking soda, chocolate chips, candied cherries, and sugar.
3. In another bowl, whisk eggs, egg substitute, and vanilla extract together.
4. Add wet ingredients to dry, and mix well.
5. Transfer dough to floured board. Roll into log and cut log in half. Roll each log into a smaller log for a total of 4.
6. Transfer logs to prepared pan. Shape into 3-inch width. Pat with hand to 1-inch thickness.
7. Set pan on middle oven rack and bake 30 minutes.
8. Remove biscotti from oven and set on cooling rack for 10 minutes. Lower oven temperature to 300 degrees.
9. Using a serrated knife, cut each log into 1/2-inch slices. Stand on pan with space between them.
10. Return to oven and bake 20 minutes. Cool thoroughly before storing.

Caregiver Tips

Humidity affects flour. If dough seems too dry, add a few drops of water. To reduce prep time, prepare the wet and dry ingredients ahead of time. Combine ingredients on baking day and finish the recipe.

PERUVIAN HOT CHOCOLATE

My husband lived in Lima, Peru when he was five years old until he was ten. His father was a physician at the British-American Hospital there. While they were in Lima, my mother-in-law learned how to make Peruvian hot chocolate. After the family returned to the States, she made it for parties. This recipe is based on an ancient Mayan drink made with cocoa beans, wine, and hot peppers. This rich, frothy brew is a dessert by itself.

Prep Time: 20 minutes
Servings: 8

Ingredients

3 squares baking chocolate
1/2 cup granulated sugar
1/8 teaspoon salt (to bring out the sweetness)
2 cups boiling water
6 cups whole milk, heated
2 teaspoons pure vanilla extract (or the seeds of 1 vanilla bean)
Whipped cream, sweetened, for garnish
Cinnamon sticks, for garnish

Method

1. Put chocolate in small saucepan and melt over low heat.
2. Stir in sugar and salt.
3. Gradually add boiling water to chocolate. Cook over medium heat 5 minutes.
4. Whisk in hot milk and vanilla. Continue whisking until hot chocolate is foamy.
5. Pour into mugs and garnish with whipped cream and a cinnamon stick.

Caregiver Tips

Mexican chocolate, the kind that looks like a hockey puck, may be used for this recipe. Peruvians whip the hot chocolate with a wooden frothing stick—available from cooking stores or online.

FRESH STRAWBERRY PIE

You can really savor the sweetness of strawberries in this fresh berry pie. Thanks to a premade crust, this pie comes together quickly.

Prep Time: 30 minutes + chilling
Servings: 8

Ingredients

2 cups strawberries, 1 cup whole and 1 cup mashed
Ready-made graham cracker crust
4 tablespoons cornstarch
1 cup granulated sugar
1/2 cup water
Half a lemon, juiced
Whipped cream or whipped topping, sugar free, for garnish

Method

1. Take leaves off whole berries and arrange in crust, large end down.

2. Combine mashed berries, cornstarch, sugar, water, and lemon juice in medium saucepan.
3. Cook over medium heat, stirring constantly, until mixture thickens.
4. Cool 10 minutes.
5. Pour over whole berries in crust.
6. Cover and refrigerate 1 hour to set.
7. Cut into slices and garnish with whipped cream or topping.

Caregiver Tips

You may also make this pie with a ready-made chocolate crust. Top with whipped cream and drizzle with chocolate sauce.

OLD-FASHIONED COCONUT SQUARES

These sweet treats are delicious and mail well. I sent them to my husband when he was in college and to my younger daughter and twin grandkids when they were in college. The original recipe comes from the *Good Housekeeping Cookbook*, published in 1955. I learned to cook from this book and, although my copy is tattered, torn, and food-stained, I treasure it. This is my version of the original recipe.

Prep Time: 25 minutes + baking
Oven Temperature: 350 degrees
Servings: 16

Ingredients
3/4 cup all-purpose flour
1/2 teaspoon baking powder
1/2 teaspoon salt
1/4 cup butter-flavored Crisco
1 large egg, room temperature
1 cup dark brown sugar
1 teaspoon pure vanilla extract

1 tablespoon orange zest

1 cup shredded coconut + 1/2 cup shredded coconut for topping

1 tablespoon butter, melted

1 tablespoon granulated sugar

Method

1. Heat oven to 350 degrees. Coat an 8" x 8" pan with cooking spray.
2. Whisk flour, baking powder, and salt together.
3. Cream Crisco, egg, brown sugar, vanilla, and orange zest together with electric mixer
4. Add dry ingredients.
5. Work 1 cup of coconut into dough.
6. Spread dough in prepared pan.
7. Combine melted butter, granulated sugar, and 1/2 cup coconut. Sprinkle over batter and bake 35 minutes.
8. Cut into squares when warm.

Caregiver Tips

For color, I decorate the top with multicolored sprinkles before baking.

ORANGE AND CINNAMON DESSERT SAUCE

This sauce turns fresh orange segments and plain cake into a special dessert. Pour the sauce over vanilla ice cream and you have the flavors of an old-fashioned popsicle—vanilla ice cream and orange sherbet.

Prep Time: 25 minutes + chilling
Servings: 6

Ingredients

1 cup fresh orange juice
6 tablespoons granulated sugar
1 small cinnamon stick
Dash salt
2 tablespoons Grand Marnier (optional)
Fresh orange segments, frozen vanilla yogurt, angel food cake, or pound cake

Method

1. Pour juice into medium saucepan. Add sugar, cinnamon stick, and salt.
2. Cook over medium heat, stirring frequently, until sauce becomes syrupy. Add Grand Marnier.
3. Chill 1 hour.
4. Serve over fresh orange segments, vanilla ice cream, angel food cake, or pound cake.

Caregiver Tips

Grand Marnier is an expensive after-dinner drink. However, you can buy a small, sample-sized bottle from the liquor store.

LUSCIOUS RASPBERRY-RICOTTA PARFAITS

A parfait is a classy ending to any meal. This combination of raspberries, Ricotta cheese, and cream cheese will please anyone.

Prep Time: 20 minutes + chilling
Servings: 6

Ingredients

1 package (9 ounces) chocolate wafers
1 pint fresh raspberries
2 tablespoons granulated sugar
1 cup Ricotta cheese (low fat or fat free)
1/2 cup (4 ounces) neufchatel cheese, with 1/3 less fat, room temperature
1/4 cup powdered sugar
1 tablespoon water
2 tablespoons whipping cream
1 teaspoon pure vanilla extract
1 carton (8 ounces) whipped topping, sugar free
Mini chocolate chips (regular or sugar free), for garnish

Method

1. Put 15 chocolate wafers in food processor and pulse to fine crumbs, or put in plastic zipper bag and crush with rolling pin.

2. Rinse berries, transfer to bowl, and sprinkle with 2 tablespoons sugar.

3. Put Ricotta and Neufchatel cheeses, powdered sugar, water, whipping cream, and vanilla extract in medium bowl. Beat with electric mixer until fluffy.

4. Spoon some chocolate crumbs into each parfait glass. Add a layer of whipped cheese mixture and top with a few raspberries. Repeat layers once.

5. Garnish with chocolate chips.

Caregiver Tips

Shortbread, almond cookies, lemon cookies, Italian amaretti, gingersnaps, and other plain cookies may be used for crumbs. Kids and grandkids may wish to assemble the desserts. Don't have any parfait glasses? Layer the desserts in jelly jars, small glasses, or clear plastic cups.

Appendix A

SODIUM FACTS

Sodium can be a health issue for caregivers and receivers alike. The human body needs salt for fluid balance and for the heart to work properly. Doctors and nutritionists recommend a minimum of 500 milligrams of sodium per day to sustain normal metabolic functioning, but the vast majority of Americans eat far more. What you think is the normal amount of sodium may really be the Upper Limit (UL). Too much sodium increases your blood pressure, a leading risk factor for heart disease and stroke.

How much sodium should you eat? For people two years and older, the amount is no more than 2,300 milligrams. For men and women age fifty-one and older, African Americans age two and older, and anyone with hypertension, diabetes, or kidney disease (no matter their age), the recommendation is 1,500 milligrams. To give you an idea of how much this is, a teaspoon of table salt equals 2,325 milligrams of sodium—more than Upper Limit levels.

Eating too much sodium is a public health problem for America. Sodium is everywhere: convenience foods, processed foods, fast-food meals, restaurant meals, bread, cheese, pizza, and other foods. To reduce sodium consumption, the Centers for Disease Control and

Prevention (CDC) created World Salt Awareness Week, which is from March 10th through the 16th.

The CDC has some recommendations:

- Read all nutrition labels carefully
- Choose the lowest-sodium foods
- Bypass processed foods that are high in sodium
- Eat more fruits and vegetables
- Use fresh ingredients to prepare meals
- Eat natural potassium (such as a banana)

The American Heart Association advises people to track their sodium intake, and has posted a Sodium Tracker on its website. (http://www.heart.org/HEARTORG/ GettingHealthy/NutritionCenter/HealthyEating/How-to-Track-Your-Sodium_UCM_449547_Article.jsp#. Vo00vvkrLIU) Table salt is about 40 percent sodium. A quarter-teaspoon of salt equals about 575 milligrams of sodium. A half-teaspoon of salt equals about 1,150 milligrams of sodium. Three-quarters of a teaspoon of salt equals about 1,725 milligrams of sodium. And one teaspoon of salt equals about 2,300 milligrams.

Mayo Clinic, in a website article, *Sodium: How to Tame Your Salt Habit*, says foods that claim to contain less sodium may not live up to the claim after you have checked the serving size. Sodium is an acquired taste, according to Mayo, and the more you consume, the more you want. Similarly, the less sodium you eat, the less you want. Cutting back on sodium consumption takes time. Eventually the craving for sodium diminishes, and this allows you "to enjoy the taste of the food itself, with heart-healthy benefits," Mayo Clinic summarizes.

I reduced the sodium in many recipes to benefit your health and your loved one's health. The meals you fix for your loved one need to be appropriate for his or her appetite. Because John is in a wheelchair, he is less active, and therefore has less appetite. Still, I kept serving him big meals, a habit left over from raising our teenage grandchildren for seven years. Fortunately, I came to my nutrition senses, and served John smaller meals. I also realized that large servings can intimidate a loved one who isn't feeling well.

There are other things to consider. Your loved one may be having chemotherapy or just finished a course of treatment. Chemotherapy can make a person feel nauseated, and take away their interest in food. The effects of your loved one's medications must also be considered. Some medicines may cause dry mouth and/or sore throat, which can be common among those who are taking many pills. Sauces, gravies, soups, juices, and flavored water can help a loved one who has a dry mouth.

Physicians and dietitians don't like to recommend salt substitutes because many contain potassium chloride, which can be harmful for those taking medications for heart failure and high blood pressure. Eating large amounts of a salt substitute can harm your loved one's health, especially if he or she has kidney problems. So you need to read product labels carefully and buy low-sodium foods. Substitute fresh or dried herbs for salt. Keep in mind that many bread products are high in salt. One of the best ways to lower the craving for salt is to take the shaker off the table. Do it today!

Appendix B

COOKING TIPS

- **Set aside one prep day a week.** Saturday or Sunday may be a good day. Once you've decided on a prep day, try to stick to this schedule.

- **Check product labels.** Ingredients are listed in order of amount, with the highest amounts first. Read every word and pay special attention to the serving size. Keep in mind that sometimes manufacturers reduce the serving size to lower the calorie count.

- **Buy store brands.** Often store brands are made by manufacturers with names you would recognize. To learn more about store brands, talk with the store manager or a department manager.

- **Make extra.** Even if you're cooking for two, make the entire recipe, and freeze some. Then, when you're short on time, you can reach in the freezer and "find" dinner.

- **Serve meatless meals twice a week.** This is a great money-saver. Although the price of eggs has gone up, they are still a bargain, and a quick meal. Pasta is also a bargain. Buy whole wheat pasta or a brand with added fiber.

- **Restock dried herbs.** Over time, dried herbs lose their flavor, and you can barely taste them. Replace herbs that have been on your shelf for more than a year.

- **Shred cheese yourself.** Preshredded cheese has a coating on it to prevent clumping. This can affect the melting property of the cheese. Shredded cheese is a handy product, but it costs more. It's wiser to buy block cheese and shred it yourself.

- **Match pan size to burner size.** A small pan on a large burner won't heat food as efficiently as a small pan on a small burner. Invest in some new pans if necessary.

- **Wash big loads of dishes at lunchtime.** By evening, you're starting to drag. The last thing you want to do is wash dishes or unload a dishwasher late at night. Doing big loads at noon gives you more time for hobbies and family activities.

- **Get a cast-iron skillet.** Teflon is wonderful, but it eventually comes off, and you may be consuming specks of it. You can avoid this problem by buying a pre-seasoned, cast-iron skillet. Follow the manufacturer's washing and re-seasoning instructions.

- **Use sharp knives and keep them sharp.** Dull knives can be dangerous. Buy a knife sharpener and use it when necessary. Store knives carefully to prevent blade damage.

- **Invest in kitchen gadgets.** Things like a turkey baster, slotted spoon, pasta fork, plastic whisk, and heat-resistant rubber scraper save you time. This alone makes them worth the investment.

- **Have different-sized storage dishes.** Whether you prefer glass or plastic, you need a variety of storage containers. Keep them in a drawer close to the fridge.

Appendix C

FOOD SAFETY

Food safety is important for all family members, but it's especially important for your loved one. Although you think you're being safe when preparing food, you may be making some mistakes. To be safe, wash your hands before you fix food, after you have prepared food, and before you touch new food. Wash your hands in warm water, lather with soap, and continue washing for at least twenty seconds. Dry your hands with a paper towel or a freshly laundered cloth one. Here are some other food safety tips:

- Wash hands again after blowing your nose, or touching your face or hair.
- Wipe counters and refrigerator door handles with disinfectant wipes.
- Launder dish cloths and towels daily.
- Use two cutting boards, one for raw meat, poultry, and seafood, and another for produce.
- Close the refrigerator and freezer doors as quickly as possible to keep cold inside.
- Use an instant-read thermometer to tell if meat or poultry are done.

- Never place cooked food on the same platter or plate that previously held raw food.
- Wash the skin of fruits, including melons, before cutting.
- Keep cold foods at 40 degrees and warm foods at 140 degrees.
- Refrigerate leftover food immediately.
- Store raw meat in a tightly sealed container.
- Store fruits and vegetables in separate refrigerator drawers.
- Set your refrigerator temperature between 32 degrees and 40 degrees.
- Set your freezer temperature to zero degrees.
- Keep a properly functioning thermometer in your refrigerator and another in your freezer.
- Microwave food only in microwave-safe containers, not just any plastic container.
- Reheat leftover gravies and sauces to boiling before serving.
- Label and date all restaurant leftovers.
- Clean garbage disposal with special tablets.
- Thaw frozen food according to manufacturer's instructions.
- Never put defrosted meat, poultry, or fish back in the freezer.

- Respect "sell by" and "use by" dates.
- Store eggs in original carton in main part of the fridge, not the door.
- Wash dishes with a cloth, not a sponge, which can be a "home" for bacteria.

Bibliography

American Heart Association. "How to Track Your Sodium." http://www.heart.org/HEARTORG/GettingHealthy/NutritionCenter/HealthyEating/How-to-Track-Your-Sodium_UCM_449547_Article.jsp#.Vo00vvkrLIU (accessed January 7, 2016).

Centers for Disease Control and Prevention. "World Salt Awareness Week: March 10–16." http://www.cdc.gov/Features/Sodium/ (accessed January 21, 2016).

Cowboys and Chuckwagon Cooking (blog). "Chuck Wagon Coffee, Just a Little History." http://cowboyandchuckwagoncooking.blogspot.com/p/chuck-wagon-coffee-just-little-history.html (accessed January 18, 2016).

Cowboys and Chuckwagon Cooking (blog). "Way of the Chuckwagon." March 25, 2010. http://cowboyandchuckwagoncooking.blogspot.com/2010/03/way-of-chuckwagon.html (accessed January 18, 2016).

Decadent Dessert Recipes. "The History of Trifle." http://www.decadentdessertrecipes.com/articles/dessert-history/the-history-of-trifle/ (accessed February 2, 2016).

Farmer, Fannie Merritt. *The Boston Cooking School Cook Book*. Boston: Little, Brown and Company, 1937, p. 160.

Good Housekeeping. *Good Housekeeping Cook Book*. New York: The Hearst Corporation, 1955, p. 475.

Hensrud, Donald D., editor. *Healthy Weight for Every Body*. Rochester, MN: Mayo Foundation for Medical Education and Research, 2005, p. 199.

Mayo Clinic. "Omega-3 in Fish: How Eating Fish Helps Your Heart," http://www.mayoclinic.org/diseases-conditions/heart-disease/in-depth/omega-3/art-20045614?pg=1 (accessed January 18, 2016).

Mayo Clinic. "Sodium: How to Tame Your Salt Habit." http://www.mayoclinic.org/healthy-lifestyle/nutrition-and-healthy-eating/in-depth/sodium/art-20045479 (accessed January 15, 2016).

National Research Council, *Dietary Reference Intakes for Water, Potassium, Sodium, Chloride, and Sulfate*. Washington, DC: National Academies Press, 2005, Chapter 6, "Sodium and Chloride," p. 269–367. http://www.nap.edu/read/10925/chapter/8#272 (accessed February 2, 2016).

1006 Summit Avenue Society, The. *Wild Rice, Star of the North: 150 Minnesota Recipes for a Gourmet Grain*. New York: McGraw-Hill Book Company, 1986, p. xiii-xviii.

Scott, Jack Denton. *The Complete Book of Pasta: An Italian Cookbook*. New York: Bantam Books, 1973, p. 14.

US Department of Agriculture Food Safety and
Inspection Service. "Danger Zone, (40°F–140°F)."
http://www.fsis.usda.gov/wps/wcm/connect/8b705ede-
f4dc-4b31-a745-836e66eeb0f4/Danger_Zone.
pdf?MOD=AJPERES (accessed January 7, 2016).

US Food and Drug Administration. "Foodborne Illness-
Causing Organisms in the U.S.: What You Need
to Know." http://www.fda.gov/downloads/Food/
FoodborneIllnessContaminants/UCM187482.pdf
(accessed January 7, 2016).

US Food and Drug Administration. "A Food Labeling
Guide: Guidance for Industry." http://www.fda.gov/
downloads/Food/GuidanceRegulation/UCM265446.pdf
(accessed February 2, 2016).

US Department of Agriculture. "All About the Vegetable
Group." ChooseMyPlate, http://www.choosemyplate.
gov/?q=vegetables (accessed January 7, 2016).

About the Author

Harriet Hodgson has been a freelance writer for 37 years, and is the author of 35 books and thousands of articles. She is a member of the Association of Health Care Journalists, a contributing writer for The Caregiver Space website, the Open to Hope Foundation website, and The Grief Toolbox website. Hodgson served on Mayo Clinic's Action on Obesity Task Force and received the Olmsted County's Lyle Weed, MD Public Health Award for leadership in "helping solve public health problems through work and service." She has appeared on more than 185 talk shows, including CBS Radio, dozens of television stations, including CNN, and given presentations at public health, Alzheimer's, and bereavement conferences. Hodgson lives in Rochester, Minnesota with her husband, John.

About the Nutrition Consultant

Frances Armstead has a Bachelor of Science degree in Nutrition, with a minor in Public Health, from the University of Minnesota. She is a Registered Dietitian (RD), Nutrition and Dietetics Technician Registered (NDTR), an active member of the Academy of Nutrition and Dietetics, and the affiliated Minnesota Academy of Nutrition and Dietetics. At home, she assists with caregiving for her father, who receives ongoing treatment for stage four colon cancer. In her spare time, Frances is a marathon runner and has completed the Twin Cities Marathon, a run of more than twenty-six miles. She is also an avid biker.

About the Photographer

Haley Earley graduated Magna Cum Laude and Phi Beta Kappa from Coe College with a Bachelor of Arts degree in Public Relations and Art. She currently works at The Salvation Army Northern Divisional Headquarters in St. Paul, MN as the Online Communications Manager and also owns her own business, Haley Earley Photography. Her exploration of photography began in middle school with her first digital camera. Shortly after receiving the camera, Haley scored first place in the Minnesota State Fair for a photo of her dog. Her college courses in black and white film, which included the lost art of the dark room, enhanced her skills. She uses photography in her day job, personal business, and many hobbies. When she is able to find a free weekend, Haley enjoys hiking with her husband, James, and their dog Phillip.

INDEX

Chocolate Dessert Waffles 209
chow mein noodles 190
coconut
    flaked 242
    macaroons 230
coffee
    beans 59
    brewed 28
    cake 123
Coffee Rub for Meat 59
collander 13
corn
    cornstarch 61, 146, 194, 226, 240
    frozen 20, 84, 128
    muffin mix 207
cloves 188
Confetti Tuna 86
Country Captain with Ground Chicken or Turkey 148
Cowboy Chili with a Jolt of Java 26
cranberries, dried 42, 49, 184, 190
crackers
    graham 240
    snack 86
    oyster 20
cream
    half and half 182
    sour 46, 132, 192, 166, 228
    whipping 111, 124, 198, 226, 238, 240, 246

US Food and Drug Administration